More than Sympathy

More than Sympathy

THE EVERYDAY NEEDS OF
SICK AND HANDICAPPED CHILDREN
AND THEIR FAMILIES

Richard Lansdown

Tavistock Publications

LONDON AND NEW YORK

First published in 1980 by
Tavistock Publications Ltd
11 New Fetter Lane, London EC4P 4EE

Published in the USA by
Tavistock Publications
in association with Methuen, Inc.
733 Third Avenue, New York, NY 10017

© 1980 Richard Lansdown

Typeset by Red Lion Setters London WC1
Printed in Great Britain by
Richard Clay (The Chaucer Press) Bungay, Suffolk

British Library Cataloguing in Publication Data

Lansdown, Richard
  More than sympathy.
  1. Family social work
  2. Handicapped children – Services for
  3. Sick children – Services for
  I. Title
  362.8'2   HV697   80-40725

  ISBN 0-422-76630-5 (Hardback)
  ISBN 0-422-76640-8 (Paperback)

To the memory of
Eve Latimer

Contents

PART FOUR

Acknowledgements

Many people have helped with the writing of this book. I would like to thank in particular: Andrew Best, whose idea it was in the first place; colleagues, parents, and children at the Hospital for Sick Children, Great Ormond Street; the representatives of many organizations for the sick and handicapped who gave up a great deal of time to answer questions; my wife, Gillian Tindall, whose comments were rarely polite and always constructive.

ILLUSTRATIONS

The author and publisher would like to thank the following for their kind permission to reproduce photographs or drawings: Express Newspapers Ltd for the drawing of Rupert and his friends (p.102); D. Collette Welch and The Muscular Dystrophy Group for the drawing of posture in Duchenne muscular dystrophy (p.182); Academic Press for the drawing from *Nadia* by Lorna Selfe (p.85); Grune & Stratton for the drawing of a spastic child from *Physically Handicapped Children* by E. Bleck and D. Nagel (p.92); Blackwell Scientific Publications Ltd for the drawing of the ear from *Clinical Anatomy* by Harold Ellis (p.112); The Royal National Institute for the Deaf for the illustration of The Standard Manual Alphabet from *Conversations with the Deaf* (p.118);

They would also like to thank Leslie A. Richardson for his kind permission to include the poem 'Muscular dystrophy' (p.186).

Introduction

This book has been written for people training to work with sick and handicapped children and their families, with particular reference to those concerned with psychological rather than medical problems. At times these problems seem as insurmountable as they are inevitable, but I have learned that with understanding the seemingly overwhelming can become bearable.

The assumptions underlying what I have written are summed up in two adages. The first is 'Forewarned is forearmed'. If one cannot anticipate what is likely to happen or what someone else is likely to say, anxiety mounts and that leads to action in which the wood cannot be seen for the trees. 'If only I had known then what I know now' is a common comment from parents, along with 'I really didn't know what to expect'.

The second adage is 'Trouble shared is trouble halved.' Parents can share much with each other and with other parents but at times they need to share also with professionals, hence the emphasis on parents as partners in both the recent British government reports on children, those of Court and Warnock. Parents know a lot about themselves and their own children. Professionals must learn to bring more than sympathy to the partnership, they must also bring knowledge.

Part One

1   The sick and the handicapped: some definitions

Nearly half the children in Britain will have been in hospital at least once by the time they are seven years old. (From the study *From Birth to Seven* by R. Davie and colleagues, 1972.)

One in five children are likely to have special educational needs at some time during their school career. (From the Report of the Warnock Committee, 1978.)

With these figures in mind a book about the problems of the sick and handicapped might be concerned with three quarters of the child population. 'Sick' can mean chronically ill with a life-threatening disease, it can mean having a heavy cold. 'Handicapped' is also used in different ways and can indicate a mild physical disability or a condition causing total loss of movement. To complicate matters further it can also refer to the degree of distress brought about by a physical condition. Definitions of what is meant by such terms are, therefore, an essential starting point to a discussion of their effects on every-day living.

SICK

Under this heading I include those children who suffer from a chronic illness which lasts over a period of years and possibly remains for life. Examples are asthma, cystic fibrosis, and leukaemia.

HANDICAPPED

In this group are those who have something organically wrong but are not, in the normally accepted use of the word, ill. Examples are cerebral palsy and mental handicap. I do not include under this heading the neurotic child, the one with a behaviour disorder or those with a learning disability.

The concept of a handicapping condition, involving a measure of the degree of distress caused by a physical condition is discussed in Chapter 3.

2   *Families*

'When I heard about my son's illness I took a crash course in Christianity but it didn't help.'

And the Lord spake unto Moses saying, Speak unto Aaron, saying, whosoever he be of thy seed . . . that hath any blemish, let him not approach to offer the bread of his God. *Leviticus*, 21, 16-17.

'The only thing I really wanted to do last night was kill both my children; I didn't think I could stand another minute of them.'

These quotations, two of which were said in my presence, may seem slanted for they illustrate only the hard side of having a sick or handicapped child and ignore the pleasure and rewards. The choice was deliberate: there are rewards, but often they are few.

One of the most fruitful recent advances in knowledge in paediatrics is the realization that the behaviour of parents is crucial to the way the child copes with his* condition. Evidence for this point was reviewed by D.T.A. Vernon in 1965 in *The Psychological Responses of Children to Hospitalisation and Illness*. This discovery, which seems so obvious today, has led to a steadily increasing amount of research into family problems.

DIFFERENCES AND SIMILARITIES: CONDITION TO CONDITION AND FAMILY TO FAMILY

Different physical conditions bring with them different sets of demands. The effects on a family of having a child born with spina bifida are by no means the same as those brought when an adolescent loses his sight. Families, too, vary enormously in

*Throughout this book I have followed the convention of referring to children in general as though they were all boys. This is to avoid the use of the cumbersome 'he or she', 'his or her', 'himself or herself', etc.

the way they react to any crisis and for the rest of this chapter I have kept differences in mind and have subdivided accordingly.

But I have been struck, not only in my reading about families but also when working with parents, by the fact that many emotions and experiences are common to a wide range of people, no matter what the child's condition may be. So as well as subdividing the chapter I have, at times, lumped everyone together when this seemed appropriate.

PROBLEMS IN THE BEGINNING

Some parents do not need to be given a diagnosis, they know as soon as they see their baby that something is wrong. Linda Wonnacott, writing in the National Children's Bureau magazine *Concern* in 1978, gave this account of those moments:

> 'Claire was born in May 1972 at home. As soon as I saw her I realised that something was very wrong. I could not believe my eyes. The features of my second child were those of a mongol. My rejection was total and complete. I just did not want to know anything about her.
>
> I thought that she was going to be a cabbage . . . a burden on my husband and myself for the rest of our lives . . . we were going to have to live with a permanent child . . . '

A radically different experience comes when a hitherto healthy child is unexpectedly taken ill. The family have vague worries that something is not right and then have a sudden, terrible shock. One family had the following experience: they were on holiday and their twelve-year-old son was lethargic and miserable. They took him to a local doctor thinking he might have some kind of bug. Within twenty-four hours they were told he had leukaemia. A measure of the extent of the shock for families like this, especially if the illness is life-threatening, is the way the date of diagnosis becomes another special anniversary: there is Christmas and birthday and the day of diagnosis day. Many parents reckon their child's life not from his birthday but from the day of diagnosis.

A common experience at the time when parents are told of their child's condition is of blanking out, of an initial failure to understand fully what is said to them. Parents may hear one word, like 'blind' or 'tumour' and then not hear anything else for the next half hour. When the booklet *Help Starts Here* was published the authors had many letters from parents asking for explanations of their child's condition. Almost certainly they had been told, but once is not enough.

Once the news has reached them, whether it is at birth or later, parents often go through several recognizable stages, similar to someone mourning a death. In a way they are mourning, for they have 'lost' a healthy child. After the initial numbness that often accompanies shock has passed, there follows for some a period of disbelief and a wild search for alternative explanations or alternative treatments. Perhaps the hospital laboratories made a mistake? Perhaps the doctor was being deliberately pessimistic to get the worst over, and the outlook is not really as bad as he said? This stage of not quite believing can go on for many years, it can pass in an hour or so.

Next, sometimes alongside disbelief and sometimes afterwards, comes anger. Parents blame their GP for not giving adequate early advice, or the hospital where the child was delivered, or their spouse for dragging them on a foreign holiday when they did not really want to go. Or they blame themselves for smoking during pregnancy or for living near a motorway.

Anger is followed by despair, the sense of an overburdening weight which will never be lifted. There is a feeling that the past will never return, the present is hell and the future can only be worse.

Finally it may all settle down, more or less, and there is a period of acceptance. This is not a time of tranquility, in which all problems are dealt with serenely and efficiently. At least it is not for most people. Rather it is one in which a sense of perspective returns, with worry being under some control.

Sometimes a stage will return, there may be a sudden flurry of anger for example. Sometimes a stage passes almost as soon as it has begun, to recur in dreams. No set times can be given for each stage or for the whole process and not all parents experience each stage as I have described it.

One group to which much of the above does not apply is those who have for long suspected that something is wrong but have not been able to convince a doctor. Out of fifty-eight cases of children with cystic fibrosis studied by Lindy Burton about a quarter were told when they first sought medical advice that they were 'fussy', 'imagining things' or 'nuts' (Burton, 1975).

For some parents like this the final diagnosis is still a shock but for others it contains an element of relief, for at last they and their child's illness are being taken seriously.

LATER PROBLEMS

Tangible problems

One of the least recognized but most pervasive facts of having a chronically sick or handicapped child is the financial burden that this entails. It is true that we have a free National Health Service but a family budget can still be diminished by mothers not being able to return to work as soon as they would have liked, or by the high cost of fares to and from hospital, or the expense of modifying a house to suit a child.

With financial demands being greater there is an increased burden on the husband to earn more. But the nature of the problem counters this, for if he does extra overtime there is always the feeling, said or unsaid, that he is escaping home difficulties by staying at work. And many fathers find they have to give up the chance of promotion because this means moving away from a trusted hospital. In one recent survey of parents of children with cystic fibrosis, one third of the fathers said that they had given up a chance of promotion because they wanted to stay near a hospital they trusted. (See Lindy Burton, *The Family Life of Sick Children*, 1975, for further examples.)

Even if there is enough money many families stop all social life once they have the responsibility of a sick or handicapped child. The reason usually given is that no one will baby sit: 'All our friends are frightened that something might happen.' I suspect that more often than not it is the parents who are frightened.

But even with the best will in the world, day to day activities of mothers of young children are limited, especially while the child cannot walk. This lack of mobility illustrates well the advantages of independence: if you have two children to look after, both of whom are heavy and unable to climb on to a bus or even step into a tube train the tendency is not go go anywhere in the first place.

Many of these problems are experienced by all parents. But normal children grow up and away. The handicapped child often stays like a baby, getting heavier and stronger all the time and the chronically sick child must, because of his dependence on medical care, remain his parents' responsibility.

Less tangible problems

An inability to predict the future

None of us can predict our future or that of our children; we can, however, say what we *think* will happen if everything in life continues as it is now. The parent of a child with a life-threatening disease can never do this, and several have told me that psychologically this is the hardest part of the whole experience. Parents feel that they cannot plan even for a summer holiday with any certainty and they cannot bear to contemplate the long-term future. One of the most poignant experiences I know is hearing a child who is likely to die within a year talk of what he will do when he is grown up.

The child with a chronic illness which is not life-threatening brings a different set of questions: will his children be affected? Will he be able to get a mortgage? Or take out life insurance? Will his illness get better or worse with time? At first these are questions the parents ask; with adolescence they are paramount in the minds of many of the children as well.

The child with a mental or physical handicap presents yet another group of questions which start from birth or from the earliest moment of diagnosis. Will he ever learn to walk? Or talk? Will he be able to go to an ordinary school? Will he manage to work? Will he be able to get married?

As a background to this uncertainty, which in itself produces chronic anxiety in a family, are two constant, nagging questions. One is hopeful: will medical science make sufficient strides in the near future to help my child? The other is despairing: what will become of him when we have gone?

Isolation

Not all parents say that they feel isolated by virtue of having a sick or handicapped child but most report a feeling that they are being pushed towards isolation. They are made to feel different, and they find that other families really do not understand or seem to want to understand what they are going through. The most common request sent to *In Touch*, a circular written for parents of the mentally handicapped, has been from parents who wish to be put in touch with others whose child has a condition similar to theirs.

This isolation comes partly from other people's attitudes. We have had little experience in our everyday lives of chronic sickness or severe handicap and so we have no framework into which to fit a sick or handicapped child when we meet one. Our ignorance leads to fear which forms a powerful barrier. As one mother rather acidly put it, 'You would think cerebral palsy was catching the way people behave.'

Partly, though, this isolation comes from the behaviour of the family itself. An enormous amount of physical and emotional energy goes into caring for many sick and handicapped children, often by night as well as by day. The result is simply that there is less time or inclination for other people. Moreover, there is often a shift in the family focus of thought. Whereas before it might have been wide-ranging, encompassing the local football team, the neighbour's roses or Aunt Mary's cats, it is now concentrated far more on the child, his treatment and his future. This was brought home to me clearly during a parents' discussion group. One father was talking about his job and he was asked if he ever thought about his sick daughter during his working day. He paused and replied, 'I never think about anything else.' Knowing this man, I realize that he did not mean that literally, but he conveyed something I have heard many other times: there is always a thought about one's child in the back of one's mind, whatever one is doing.

Guilt

This is a slippery subject, hard to define exactly, difficult to discuss with parents until one knows them well, and even then not easy to pin down. A simple theory says that all parents of sick or handicapped children feel guilty either at having produced a congenitally handicapped child or at having been so negligent as to permit a child to become ill. I have heard students talk glibly about 'maternal guilt' as though it were always present and they, the students, had a mission to uncover it.

Against this is the view that such a theory is grossly

exaggerated, being based only on a few parents who give a false impression of the total. As the Birmingham psychiatrist A.I. Roith has put it ' . . . one psychiatrist states that if parents place their child in a hospital they will feel guilty because unconsciously this means that they are trying to get rid of him. Whereas another psychiatrist has maintained that if parents keep their child at home they will have guilt feelings because they are depriving it of the best medical and nursing care!' If you look hard enough for guilt it is, indeed, not difficult to find. The truth is probably somewhere between the two views. Ronald Mac Keith, a paediatrician, said that he thought that feelings of guilt existed but they were 'probably less common than many writers state'. It seems likely that they do occur in four situations:

1. When the child's condition is known to be inherited and the parents suspected there was a risk but did nothing to find out more. Lindy Burton quotes the father of a child with cystic fibrosis: 'My first reaction on being told was to remember that my mother had told me two cousins had died of it, and I blamed myself for not thinking of it.'

2. When mothers have continued to smoke, drink heavily, or take drugs during pregnancy.

3. When parents have delayed seeking medical help at the first indication of abnormal behaviour.

4. When parents feel that they are not doing the utmost possible for their child, either in terms of obtaining the best medical care or by ensuring that social and educational provisions are as perfect as can be.

Revulsion, anger, and a feeling that it is all too much

This is not the same as the period of anger that some parents experience on being told a diagnosis. Rather it is a reaction to a specific situation, or series of situations, which wells up and threatens to become uncontrollable. I am thinking of the mother I met recently who had already lost two boys; I had to tell her that her third child was mentally handicapped. I am thinking of the unmarried mother of two boys under five, both handicapped, neither of whom would ever be able to walk. I am thinking of the mother of a child born with an ugly blemish over her left eye whose husband left her the day the girl was born. These are the parents who feel sometimes revolted by their children's inadequacies, sometimes incapable of carrying on for another hour. These feelings are not 'unnatural' as an unthinking observer might imagine; they are common, biologically normal, and have to be faced.

Indulgence and overprotection

'How can you possibly punish him, he's got cancer.' This was not said by a parent, I heard it from a friend of the parents who was commenting on how hard the mother was. But it could easily have come from a parent, for many find it quite impossible to discipline a sick or handicapped child as they do one who is normal. The result is often very unhappy little boys or girls, who do not enjoy a life when they always get their own way, who have tantrums when others thwart them, and who receive the message that even in naughtiness they are different from other children. (See Chapter 5 for a discussion on management.)

Overprotection comes even more easily and leads to parents keeping their children much younger than they need. I have heard of a mother continuing to bath a ten-year-old quite unnecessarily, because he had been born prematurely.

There are several causes of both indulgence and over-protection. Parents may feel guilty and try to compensate. They may be fearful of the child doing anything new because the old is nice and secure and the new is unknown and dangerous. They might have started by exercising reasonable care, which got out of hand because the child did not develop as others and so the parents had no guidelines. They may have deep feelings of which they are not fully aware which make them want to keep the child a baby, for it is acceptable to have a totally dependent baby and so it feels more comfortable to pretend really that there is nothing wrong with the child, only that he is still young.

How much information to give to the child

For some children the question does not arise. The profoundly mentally handicapped may not learn to understand any information about his condition. The child with diabetes must have explanations given in order to keep him alive. But three kinds of problem do come frequently.

The first is how to explain to a very young child why he cannot do what others can. 'Why can't I use my hands, mummy?'

The second is to decide how much to tell a child with a possibly incurable, life-threatening disease. Children under the age of six or so are thought to have only a hazy understanding of death, but even if this is accepted, what about the period after six? (For a further discussion of children's concepts of death see Chapter 18.)

The third problem is related to the second and is whether to tell the child the actual name of his complaint, an especially difficult task if it is a fearful name like cancer.

Denying the illness

Some families do, from time to time, play with the idea that there is really nothing wrong with their child. These are parents of children who for long periods seem quite well. They look healthy, run around with their friends, eat and sleep well, and get on well at school. At times like this some parents even stop the child's treatment. They usually start again quite quickly when the child goes into relapse.

Some families accept a physical diagnosis but stubbornly refuse to believe what they are told about a child's mental state. No matter how many tests are given they always find an excuse: the child is shy, doesn't like hospitals or clinics, has a cold, had a cold last week, is lazy, playing everyone up . . . Sooner or later they have to come to terms with the extent of the handicap, and very hard it can be.

Brothers and sisters

By the time they are eleven, five out of six children have a brother or sister. Nearly all children who have siblings spend more time with them than they do with their father, and once they are ten they see more of their siblings than they do of their mother. In the last few years there has been a slow accumulation of knowledge about the siblings of sick and handicapped children, most of it gained from interviews with their parents. (See Stephen Kew, *Handicap and Family Crisis*, 1975, for a review of this work.)

The birth of a normal brother or sister in a normal family can bring jealousy and a return to much younger behaviour. Some children start to wet the bed again, or demand to be fed from a bottle, or even stop talking. One study of a series of children suggested that over half were disturbed, to some extent, by the arrival of another child. (See Dora Black and Claire Sturge, *The Young Child and his Siblings*, 1979.) It is not surprising, then, that the birth of a handicapped child, or one who is clearly sick, or the development of an illness in a hitherto well child, can lead to problems, for there is often a shift in the family balance as well as an accentuation of jealousy.

The shift comes with parents having to devote much time and energy to the sick or handicapped child. At the same time, the well child is often left to live up to all his parents' expectations; he now has to achieve for two.

Summarizing what we do know of siblings and their problems the following points emerge:

1. Children who are younger than the patient are generally more vulnerable than those who are older. This is probably due to a decrease in attention often given to younger, healthy children.

2. Girls are more vulnerable than boys, perhaps because they are seen as substitute mothers.

3. The most powerful effects come from inherited and life-threatening conditions, e.g. muscular dystrophy, rather than chronic, non-fatal conditions like cerebral palsy. Children fear that they, or their children, might develop the former and they are often given far too little information to help to allay such fears.

4. A major problem comes when one child has a degenerative condition and then a sibling develops the same condition and can anticipate what will happen to him. Margaret Atkin, a social worker who has helped many such families, quotes Dryden to illustrate this point:

> *With unerring doom*
> *He sees what is, and was, and is to come.*

5. There is no characteristic disorder evident in siblings, but attention-seeking behaviour, jealousy, and regression to an earlier stage can all be expected.

6. About one third of the siblings of sick and handicapped

children can be expected to show some disturbance. Others, though, seem to blossom and are reported to develop a tender protectiveness towards the sick child.

7. Sometimes children can be loving and protective towards a handicapped child within the family, but find themselves overcome with embarrassment when they are out in public with him. Sometimes they are teased at school and may be reluctant to bring friends home.

This might have given a gloomy impression. In fact one can look at the figures less pessimistically: about two thirds of the brothers and sisters who have been studied have shown themselves able to cope without showing undue strain.

Grandparents

As a group we know little about grandparents; they have received far less attention from research workers than parents or siblings. They can be a powerful ally to parents, providing comfort and understanding and sometimes practical help, either financially or by baby sitting. They can, on the other hand, be damaging to the whole family. There is the grandparent who resolutely refuses to believe that anything is wrong with the child and cannot understand why his name is not down for the family public school. There is the grandparent who sends birthday and Christmas presents to everyone in the family except the handicapped child. There is the one who mutters about there being 'nothing of that sort of thing on our side'. But our information on them comes from individual accounts, a large-scale family based survey examining their influence is overdue.

Little things

Some years ago I visited a large house with a big, overgrown garden. The people who owned the house were keen on gardening and I was surprised to see roses with dead heads on them. Then I reflected on the fact that this family included two handicapped children, one of whom was autistic and had to be watched all day. There just was not time for gardening, or if time had been made then something else would have gone. Up to a point this is so with any family with small children. As I have noted already, the handicapped child often stays, in behaviour, small for years and years. It is little things that gradually wear parents down and yet they receive hardly any attention from commentators or researchers.

Communication with professionals

In 1970 Sheila Hewett published *The Family and the Handicapped Child*. She wrote then:

> 'There is one central theme which runs like a thread through the various sections of this report: briefly it is clear that the channels of communication between the parents themselves and those who have the responsibility of trying to help them are constricted and congested at very many different points.'

Over ten years later the picture was similar, as the Warnock Committee on Special Education noted. Parents still find themselves in a jungle of professionals and it is little wonder that they often feel they are battling against them all. The Warnock Committee recommended that one Named Person be responsible for co-ordinating work. The need is undoubted, not only to help parents in their communication with professionals but to help professionals communicate with each other.

Parental health

Overall conclusions on this topic cannot be made because there is such variation between families. But there is a tendency for parents of handicapped children, especially the mentally handicapped, to have higher than normal rates of ill health, both physical and mental. If the family is in poor housing, without adequate community support, the likelihood of ill health is even greater. (See D. Pilling's *The Handicapped Child*: *Research Review*, Vol. 3, 1973.)

The marriage

A consideration of the effects of stress on the state of the marriage really should include everything that has been said in this chapter up to this point. An assumption is often made that because 'a handicapped child means a handicapped family' all marriages are in danger of imminent collapse.

No one denies that there is an additional strain imposed on any family, and several researchers have tried to see if any particular type of condition in a child brings a greater divorce rate than is present in the rest of the population. So far such studies have not shown that divorce is more common among parents of either sick or handicapped children. What has been shown, though, is that parents who have been married for at least five years and who have normal older children have a better record of coping than others. (See D. Pilling, *The Child with Spina Bifida*, 1973.) If we move away from surveys to what individual parents say the consistency is striking. In my experience almost all say that good marriages are made better and bad ones worse.

COPING

By 'coping' I do not mean eliminating all difficulties; that is impossible. Instead I follow the ideas of the psychologist Stephen Kew, who saw it as being a matter of organizing one's life in such a way that problems can be overcome, without the rest of one's life being constantly interfered with.

The factors that seem to be present in a family that copes are:

1. An understanding of the child's condition and his future.

2. An understanding of the needs of other members of the family.

3. The reduction as far as possible of the sense that the sick or handicapped child is dependent on one or all other family members.

4. A feeling that they, the family members, are able to contribute to their child's wellbeing in a way that extends beyond just taking day to day care of him.

At diagnosis

The key word here is *time*. There are many horror stories of brusque doctors giving a hurried opinion to parents and sending them away to puzzle and to grieve. A sizeable minority of one group of parents of children with spina bifida said they had never really had the condition explained to them. This may or may not be true; none of us has a perfect memory and parents often feel angry at the person who first brings bad news. It is helpful, though, to give parents a chance for a second interview, a few days after the first, when they can ask questions, for they are often too distraught to do this the first time round. I have heard of one doctor who tape records all his first interviews and lends the tape to the parents.

Some parents are given a booklet, usually published by one of the voluntary societies, explaining their child's condition in non-technical language. Sometimes they are helpful but I have found some of them rather over-optimistic. If they are worried the parents should be given a chance to discuss the contents with their doctor a little while later when they have had time to digest them. The comments in them can then be related to their own child.

A dilemma that some doctors find themselves in is when to give the news, an especially difficult point if the mother is weak from childbirth, and whether to insist on telling both parents at once. On these subjects I can write only from what several parents have said rather than from research studies. The answers that emerge seem to point in the direction of their wanting to be told as soon as possible, certainly within a few hours of the doctor knowing. No agreed opinion exists on the second point, some parents prefer always to be told everything together, others always insist on being separate if possible.

A full understanding of the condition implies a need to know of practical ways of helping the child and of overcoming some of the physical and financial burdens that have been mentioned in the first part of this chapter. Practical help to a family at this time can take such forms as advice on feeding to the mother of a child with a cleft lip and palate, or information about the way a blind child behaves when he hears his parents' voices, or it can be little more at first than a list of useful addresses where parents can seek help themselves. Whatever else follows in the shape of counselling and psychological support, the practical must come first.

The best person to offer this help will vary according to the nature of the problem and where the family lives. Health visitors and social workers can be helpful if they have either training or experience. If they have neither they are of little value. I heard of one health visitor who, on a visit to the mother of a child with a cleft lip, took one look at the baby and burst into tears.

Some areas, e.g. Southend and Hereford, have organized a flying squad approach so that parents of a newly diagnosed handicapped child can be visited within a couple of days by another parent. A similar service is offered for bereaved parents by the Society of Compassionate Friends. It is too early yet to comment on the general effect of this type of help but first impressions suggest that it can be most valuable.

In later years

Later, more specific help will be needed. The Royal National Institute for the Blind has a team of education advisers who visit homes, and several local authorities and at least one voluntary organization have a scheme to provide home-based educational advice to the parents of handicapped pre-school children. Other agencies, for example the Hester Adrian Centre in Manchester, run groups for parents with a focus on management. There is ample room for an expansion of all these services.

A vital piece of practical help is allowing parents to have a break from the constant demands of caring. This is true no matter what the child's problem. A break may be no more than an evening at the cinema, it may be a week in the West Indies. This opportunity can be taken only when parents have come to see that their child is not totally dependent on them, and this in itself may be something that they have to work towards. Once it has been achieved, with neighbours, grandparents, sisters, Social Services Department, or a hospital helping to care for the child, parental anxiety will decrease, for until that moment there will always be a feeling of dread lest anything should happen to the parents. The anxiety about the long-term future may remain, but the acute worry will pass and this will be of certain value to the child himself.

Another way of getting if not a break at least some help with care is through the scheme of Community Service Volunteers. These people, generally young, work for a specific period on a specific project which can include helping in a family for a few weeks or a few months.

Anxiety about the present, future, and sometimes the past has to be faced. A parent who cannot cope with worries will not cope with his child either, indeed he will more likely than not transmit them to the child. Some parents find talking to a neighbour a lifesaving activity; others seek help from a social worker or, more rarely in my experience, from their GP. Some find meeting other parents in a group to be a good way of both learning and of sharing problems. Ideally a wide range of provision should be available in the community where the family lives; in practice such help is sparse and scattered.

One of the aims of psychological support of this nature is to increase both a family's awareness of each other's needs and their ability to talk about them. I have heard on more than one occasion one of a couple say, in a parents' group, 'I've never told anyone this, not even my wife'. This all needs time, though, and the parent must feel confidence in the person or people he is talking with. It is a great mistake for anyone to expect to help in anything but a superficial way until the necessary trust has been built up, and that can take months or even years.

Religious faith is always tested, and sometimes sought, immediately after a diagnosis of a serious condition. Some people find comfort in the thought that God has chosen them to look after this particular child, others wonder why God has punished them so. Some say that without their faith they could not continue living, others say they lost all faith on the day of the child's diagnosis.

There is one vital aspect of long-term psychological support, no matter who gives it, and that is the need to know that there is always someone, readily accessible, to whom one can turn in a time of crisis. I know one father who had no one. He and his wife could not talk properly to each other because she could not bear to face the possibility of their child's death. He worked all day and could not easily get to a hospital to meet social workers, and for various reasons he had not been helped locally. Then one day he wrote to a faith healer and an intermittent correspondence was set up. This, according to the man himself, saved his sanity. He never met the healer and is not convinced that his son was helped by him, but he did have a person to get in touch with when everything was getting him down.

A summary of work done in various fields can be found in Janet Carr's annotation *Handicapped Children*: *Counselling the Parents* (1970) and in Robert Noland's *Counselling Parents of the Mentally Retarded* (1970).

GIVING INFORMATION TO CHILDREN

As I noted above, difficult decisions fall into two groups. The first is explaining the cause of a disability to a child or his siblings, or to other children who are curious. 'You can't walk properly because you were born with something wrong with your legs' or 'because your legs don't work as well as other people's' is the best that I have known parents come up with when talking to young children. It is helpful to follow this up with some reassurance that other parts of the body do work well. As children gain in understanding, so it is possible to give them more detailed medical information, not forgetting a short intro-duction to genetics, especially for siblings.

Much harder is the problem of what to do with information that carries an emotional charge to the parents. Should a child with cystic fibrosis be told about impotence, should a child with leukaemia be given the name of the disease?

Most parents say that they tell children as much as the child can cope with, but I sometimes think that what they really mean is that they tell as much as they, the parents, can cope with telling. If one knows the parents well it sometimes helps to rephrase the question to allow them to ask themselves what is being risked by not giving full information. In particular, the following points can be discussed:

If information is withheld, and the child discovers it from another source, how will he then feel about his parents? Will he continue to trust them?

Will the strain of keeping something from him lead to greater problems than those that might arise if he knew?

Is there a hidden message being conveyed by secrecy? If there is, perhaps the hidden message is that there is something shameful about his illness.

Do children not pick up half truths from what they overhear? If so, is it not better that they hear the full truth?

Reading these points may give the impression that I am wholly in favour of telling all children everything. While I do tend in the direction of giving as much information as possible to children, I do acknowledge that there are times, for example when a child is facing death, when a powerful drive exists on the part of both parents and child not to share this kind of knowledge. This is not the same as saying that children should not know; it is arguing that parents may not be the best people always to discuss such matters. At times like this I rely on the formula that is sometimes an easy way out but sometimes applies: it all depends on the child and his family.

SOME CONCLUDING, MISCELLANEOUS POINTS

I suggest that parents:

1. Develop a formula for explaining their child's condition to strangers. This is something that has to be done time and time again and having a set pattern is a help.

2. Actively help the handicapped child establish relationships with other children. Once a friendship has been set up children stop noticing the handicap.

3. In general, tell the child as much about his condition as he, and the parents, can cope with, not forgetting that information has to be updated as the child gets older.

4. Tell siblings no more than the sick or handicapped child has been told, unless he is mentally handicapped and can understand little. This is especially important for children with a life-threatening disease. For some siblings a book may be useful: for example, Harriet Langsam Sobol's *My Brother Stephen is Retarded* (1978). (See page 206 for a note of other books, dealing with other conditions, which have been specially written for children.)

5. Be aware of the dangers of neglecting each other.

6. Tell at least one work colleague of the child's condition. If a crisis arises work relationships are then much easier.

7. Make sure that the child's class teacher knows of the nature of the child's condition.

I suggest that those working with parents:

1. Never say 'Don't worry'. Parents will and should worry at times. It is better to try to stop them worrying all the time.

2. Never say 'I know how you feel'; that is, unless you really do.

3. Never underestimate the value of listening but remember that parents must trust you before they will talk. To expect them to pour out their heart at first meeting is naive.

4. Always ask yourself what practical help you can provide.

3   Perceptions: how we see children and how they see themselves

'Daddy, why is everyone staring at me?'
'Sweetheart, you've just got to learn to stare right back.'

'What I really love doing is going out shopping on my own. For a whole hour I am relaxed; I don't have to worry and wonder what people are going to say.'

Parents, and sometimes children, plead to be left alone, to be treated as normal human beings. This is a fair request but we cannot avoid the fact that handicapped and seriously sick children are, indeed, abnormal, and to expect society to take no notice is unrealistic. It is true that some people can successfully pretend to ignore the unusual but most show any or all of the following reactions:

Curiosity. We are all curious. As children we needed the drive to find out about our world, and the need continues to be part of our adult make up. It is not surprising that people stare at an unusual sight, even in public. I remember taking two girls on a visit to a stately home; one was blind and the other spastic. Our progress through the house and gardens was accompanied by a series of swivelling heads. This level of curiosity is bearable, it becomes offensive when it shades into prolonged staring or impertinent questions.

Pity. The amount of pity shown towards anyone depends on the extent to which the observer is able to identify with the other person. A classic comparison is between the blind and the deaf. The blind excite more pity, as can be judged partly by comparison of the money received by charities, because it is far easier to close one's eyes than it is to close one's ears. The result is that many people imagine that blindness is the more severe handicap. In contrast to this many workers in the field argue that the isolating nature of hearing loss makes it psychologically more stressful.

Repulsion. Some people cannot bear to look at the disfigured, others cannot bring themselves to think of a child who is crippled. In both cases the mainspring of the emotion is the same: it is a revulsion against the abnormal, a feeling which has deep roots in human history. In Ancient Greece the handicapped child was exposed on a hillside to die, for he was seen as a potentially intolerable burden to others. The need to reject the deviant in order to maintain care for the healthy may strike us as reprehensible; it is biologically normal.

Fear. The 'fear of the unknown' is commonly recognized. It leads some people to fear any child who is removed from their immediate experience, and for many that includes almost all the children discussed in this book. The mechanism behind the fear seems to be related to the difficulty that is experienced in trying to anticipate what an unknown quantity will do or say.

THE CONCEPT OF STIGMA

It is hard, but possible, for a person who is different to come to terms with expressions of curiosity, pity, repulsion, and fear, for they are all readily understood. Much less easy is the feeling of being ostracized for what one appears to be rather than for what one is. This is the feeling of being stigmatized. The word stigma was originally used by the Greeks to refer to bodily signs burnt or cut into the body to indicate that the person was unusual or bad. The crucial element in the concept is not just that of being singled out, it is not even that of rejection, it is the assumption that the person who looks very different is in some way morally inferior to those who are normal. This is exemplified in Shakespeare's portrayal of Richard III as 'disnatured', his mis-shapen body being the outward manifestation of a distorted mind. (For a full discussion of stigma see Erving Goffman's book of that name, published in 1963.)

CHANGES IN PERCEPTION

Attitudes do not remain constant. For example, Ancient Hebrew texts suggest that the writers regarded mental illness in a more tolerant light than is the case today. In Medieval Europe abnormal children were often thought to be changelings, that is babies left by fairies in the place of human children, and therefore, possibly, bringers of good fortune. (See Gillian Tindall, *A Handbook on Witches*, 1965.) By the nineteenth century the mentally handicapped child was likely to be perceived as evil, as one who has been punished by God.

Variations between cultures can be observed as well. In Britain and America the fat child has been shown to be less acceptable to other children than those with a physical disability; in Holland obesity seems to be perceived differently, as I discovered when a Dutch student of mine replicated the American work and found that fat children were ranked in the middle range of acceptability. Anyone interested in following up this area of research should look at the paper on 'Handicap, appearance and stigma' by S.A. Richardson (1971).

Attitudes towards a crippled child vary from country to country as well, as is discussed in Robert Scott's chapter in a book edited by J. Douglas, *Deviance and Respectability* (1970).

PERCEPTIONS AND KNOWLEDGE

As a general rule of thumb, the more an observer knows about a condition, the less likely he is to come out with an insensitive comment. The more we know, the less we fear and the more we can see through to the normal bits of the person underneath.

For example, most people know that diabetes is something to do with too much sugar in the body, or is it too little? Anyway, it is something like that and it is treated with injections and we all know about them so it is not too fearful. At least it is not fearful compared to epilepsy, which means fits and having something wrong with your brain and thrashing around and frothing at the mouth. No matter that the person who thinks that may never have seen a fit, what counts is that those are his thoughts.

But it is not as simple as that. There are times when ignorance can bring complacency. Cystic fibrosis, for example, may arouse little emotion because it can easily be confused with fibrositis and thought not to be very serious.

THE CHILD'S SELF CONCEPT

From the time we become aware of ourselves as separate individuals we build up a picture of ourselves in our minds. We learn that we are clever or stupid, ugly or beautiful, strong or weak. We learn from the way others behave, from what they say and from how they look. And we go on learning all the time right into adulthood.

As the child's self concept develops so comes a perception of psychological needs, although few children could put them into words. Margaret Donaldson, in *Children's Minds* (1978), has argued that children need to feel effective, competent and independent. There is irony in this when we think of sick or handicapped children, for they are rarely totally independent, often incompetent and seldom fully effective as they would have been had it not been for their physical difficulties.

The realization of failure to gain one or all of these three reaches children in different ways and at different times. At first everyone thinks himself to be normal, like the partially sighted child who, when given glasses for the first time, was astonished at the clarity of the picture on a television set; he had imagined that everyone saw as he had. Sooner or later they learn that they are different. They may still see themselves as loved and wanted by their families, but they become aware that one or more of the three needs are not being met. At that moment they become psychologically vulnerable.

The acquisition of a sense of difference and hence of vulnerability is an example of a way in which all the children described in this book are, to some extent similar and yet cannot all be lumped together in all ways. Although the vulnerability may be something held in common, there is a difference between the child who is born with a certain condition and one who develops one in later life, well after his self concept has begun to develop.

The families of children with a congenital handicap often try to shield the child from the world. They provide what Goffman has called 'a protective capsule'. At first only positive messages of normality and acceptance are given, so that the child may spend the first few years of life building up a picture of himself as both valued and normal. Gradually, and in what is hoped will be a carefully controlled way, information about his condition is allowed to filter through. This is a strategy that can be successful but the capsule is difficult to maintain, especially when there is a major change in the child's circumstances, such as going to a new school or moving to a new neighbourhood. The capsule can then be shattered.

On the other hand, the child who acquires a problem almost invariably does so suddenly and the result is a sense of confusion.

> 'Suddenly I woke up one morning and found that I could not stand . . . Something had happened and I became a stranger . . . Even my dreams did not know me. They did not know what they ought to let me do.' (N. Linduska, *My Polio Past*, 1947)

MEASURING DISTRESS

It is no use to try to estimate psychological distress from medical measures. Indeed, such measures may be misleading, for it is not true that the more severe physical problem is always harder to bear than the lesser. The severely afflicted person does at least have the advantage of knowing where he stands *vis-à-vis* the rest of the world; he and his family learn to anticipate the responses of others. The mildly afflicted often find themselves in situations when they cannot do this, or they find that they are treated differently at different times of day. An example is the child with a mild visual handicap who may receive sympathy when he has to hold a book close to his eyes and derision when he cannot catch a ball.

Psychological classification should rather be based on the functional effect of the condition on the child and his family, that is on the way in which everyday life has been affected. One way of classifying with functional effects in mind has been devised by a group of workers at Bedford College, London University. (See the Open University course book, *The Handicapped Person in the Community*, 1974, for more details.)

Three groups have been distinguished in this system:

The first consists of the impaired. An impairment is any physical loss or defect, no matter how slight.

The second group is the disabled. A disablement is an impairment which leads to a person being unable to carry out certain activities that are considered, in his family, to be normal.

The third group is the handicapped, that is those whose impairment not only stops them from leading a normal life but also leads to a sense of being disadvantaged.

To illustrate the differences between these three: a child who has lost a finger will be impaired but may not be disabled. If he comes from a family where everyone plays the piano he will be disabled but he may not see this as a personal disadvantage (he may not like the piano). If, on the other hand, he is a good musician who would have been a good pianist, the loss of a finger will be a handicap.

WAYS OF HELPING

Public education can bring about a change in attitude but it is futile to imagine that society will alter overnight. People will continue to be insensitive and to overgeneralize from one aspect of abnormality to think that one defect implies a dozen others. Work aimed at helping must, therefore, be directed mainly at individual children and families, at least by most of us in the field, with the aim of helping them to cope.

A primary task is encouraging everyone concerned to distinguish between aspects of a child which are normal and those which are not. A boy with cerebral palsy, for example, will probably find it difficult to learn maths, not because he is lazy, stupid, or awkward but because of the effect of the condition on the way the brain works. Allowances should be made for this. In other ways the same child may be quite normal, for example in a desire to stay up late to watch television, and at times like that he should be treated as would any other boy.

One way of helping the maintainance of a sense of normality is by keeping in contact with the world outside the immediate family, the hospital, and the special school. It is very easy, and comfortable, to slip into a world where the normal are seen as the deviant.

Linking both points just made is the need for parents and all other adults who have anything to do with the child to be as open and honest as possible about the causes and nature of his condition. The problem of what to tell children has been discussed in Chapter 2. Let me repeat: the more that is hidden the greater the implication there is that something is shameful.

To end on an optimistic note: the girl quoted at the beginning of this chapter, who asked why everyone was staring at her, was helped to understand why and was helped to stare back. The world did not just stare, it talked back to her, and while her life has been hard she is now seen as a person in her own right.

4 Children in hospital

'He won't have a drink, he won't have a cuddle, he only wants mummy. So I've told him she's not here and he'd just better shut up.'

A five-year-old child: 'Hospital is a place where they snatch you up and hurt you.'

PSYCHOLOGICAL DAMAGE

There are times when a psychological theory catches fire and spreads throughout a country, a continent, to half the world. Although few people read the original research reports, or even the original discussions, most have some notion of what is in them. One such theory is that which asserts that a young child will suffer grave psychological damage if separated from his mother. It is this theory which underpins many of the statements made about the psychological effects of going into hospital.

The idea is not new. Indeed, in the eighteenth century it was put forward as an argument against the building of a special hospital for children. As one physician of the time put it:

'It will be apparent to any thinking person that if you take a sick child away from its mother or its nurse you break its heart at once.'

But such concepts became buried beneath the seemingly more pressing demands of medical care, and children's hospitals were built, children were taken away from parents and nannies and it was not until the work of Edelston in America and Bowlby and Robertson in Britain – work which started in the mid-1940s and still continues – that most modern thinking people returned, as a matter of principle, to the idea that hearts can be broken in hospital as well as mended.

The eighteenth-century physician, though, was writing about sick children. Recent theory, especially the work of John

Bowlby, has been concerned with the physically well. This is one example of the way in which a theory is rarely as simple as it seems; it is essential to consider not only the basic idea but some subsidiary ideas as well.

THE BASIC IDEA: ATTACHMENT AND BONDING

Babies are born helpless. Biologically they are totally dependent on an older person, mother or mother substitute, to keep them alive. For the first few months their only weapons are a cry and a smile. By six or seven months they appear to have matured sufficiently to use both these weapons in a two-way relationship with their caretakers and attachments are formed. 'Attachment' means what it says: a strong, dependent relationship. The cry is now used more selectively, e.g. when the loved person leaves, and the smile becomes a special welcome for the return.

The second part of the theory is to do with the development of more selective attachments known as 'bonds'. Bonding, the formation of special and very deep attachments, seems to be related most of all to the intensity of the relationship. Thus in Israel, where some babies pass most of the day with a nursery worker, the primary bond is still often with the mother because she plays with her children, with great attention, for a couple of hours a day.

Bowlby, in his *Child Care and the Growth of Love* (1951), has summed up the characteristics of this relationship as 'warm, intimate and continuous . . . in which both find satisfaction and enjoyment'.

Many references are made to mother-child bonds but there is little evidence that this is the only one that can be formed. If a child has an opportunity to establish relationships with a neighbour, grandparents, or nanny then multiple bonding is possible. Even if there is only one main attachment this is not always with the child's mother: one study of eighteen-month-olds showed that in nearly one third of the cases it was with the father. (See Michael Rutter, *Maternal Deprivation Reassessed*, 1972.)

Now for the central part of the theory as far as we are concerned. During the period from about six months to four or five years a bond must first of all be formed and then permanently maintained if the child is to stay psychologically secure. If the attachment pattern is perceived by the child as having been broken, i.e. if the important figure or figures in the child's life are seen to have disappeared, then he will feel rejected and vulnerable. If the break in relationships lasts, the psychological damage deepens. The age of four or five as an upper limit is deliberately vague since part of the theory rests on the fact that children are distressed when their attachment is broken because they cannot understand why this has happened. After this age most children have developed enough to understand at least in outline why they need to be separated.

This, then, is the basic idea. It has been widely quoted and widely misunderstood. It does not mean that a mother should spend every minute of every day with her child until he goes to school; it does not mean that nursery schools are evil. It *does* mean that children should spend most of their time, especially when they are feeling ill, with someone they know and can trust.

SUBSIDIARY IDEAS WHICH MAY ALSO EXPLAIN DISTRESS

Many children feel ill when they are admitted to hospital, others feel well when they go in but soon feel ill from what is done to them. This has led some authorities to question the suggestion that separation in itself is harmful. They see the child's distress as being related to his illness. As one doctor put it twenty years ago, 'None of us is quite so sweet tempered in convalescence as before an illness.'

'Hospitals are where they hurt you.' The younger the child the more he resents what is done to make him better. Perhaps we should look at finger pricks, injections, strange diets, and humiliating toilet procedures to explain why children are upset. Perhaps, but the equation is not simple: a report by D.T.A. Vernon and colleagues (1966) suggested that for children people are more important than pain.

Hospitals are dehumanized. There is a seemingly constant change of staff, each one doing a single job. One four-year-old child was observed to come into contact with twenty-five different people in three hours (R. Lindheim and colleagues, 1972). This does not happen in all hospitals but when it does it produces an effect which is the exact opposite of attachment.

The child feels he is being punished. To a young child parents are all powerful. It follows, then, that if he is in hospital with all those nasty things happening to him, he has been punished.

After all, it was his parents who brought him in the first place. This is a fair point, but it does not provide an argument against parental contact, rather it underlines the need for parents to maintain a close link with their child, to offset the sense that he might have that they have withdrawn their love.

Hospital is boring. Many wards have playleaders, many have nurses who understand both play and children. But the study published by Stacey in 1970 pointed out that some children spend up to 80 per cent of their time unattended and without occupation.

Hospitalization leads to a withdrawal of previously gained independence. At about the age of two years children begin to assert their independence and not for nothing is this period known as the 'terrible twos'. They insist on rituals before bed, or on eating only certain foods and generally play up. In hospital their independence is taken from them, hence the tantrums and returns to babyhood.

Let us now look at a composite child. Here he is, two-and-a-half years old, and he is sitting in an undignified position on a potty, just as he has learnt to use a proper lavatory. His leg hurts from an injection, and the nurse had said that it would not hurt, his eye is bandaged, and he had to eat pink blancmange for tea, and he hates the pink sort. His mother and father have gone home to his sister and he is being looked after by a nurse he has never seen before. He does not really understand why he is in hospital and he has tried crying but no one took any notice and he is fed up. One would be hard put to decide which is the main reason for his distress.

CHILDREN'S BEHAVIOUR: IN HOSPITAL AND AFTERWARDS

Moving from theory to practice, we can now examine what actually happens, how children behave first when they are in hospital and then when they return home. (The problems of long-stay children, who go home seldom or not at all, are not the subject of this book.) Not all children are obviously upset. One American writer has argued that most children will manage quite well when separated from their parents if there are other children and a television on the ward. Others have said that some children are relieved to get away from their parents' domination. It is important to remember that different people can have quite different interpretations of the same event: a quiet child is happy to one observer, depressed to another.

John Bowlby and James Robertson have proposed that three stages characterize a young child's behaviour during separation. The three stages are protest, despair, detachment.

Protest. At first the child cries, shrieks, and shows signs of doing everything in his power to change what has happened. This is seen as the period of anxiety at parental loss, or it may be that he is just cross at being in a strange place. No one, however, denies that he is upset.

Despair. Next he becomes quiet, very quiet. He may cry monotonously, he makes few demands on his environment. To some observers this is a period of deep mourning for a loved one, to others it is a time of settling down.

Detachment. He plays cheerfully, is easy to manage and accepts care from any nursing staff. He may pay little attention to his parents when they visit and is not upset when they leave. To some this means that he has given up his attachment and the psychological damage is deepening. To others, it indicates that he is happy in hospital and the nursing staff should be left alone to look after him.

There is no general agreement about the length of time that each stage may take, protest may last for an hour or a week and it may be six months before an advanced stage of detachment is reached. There is not even general agreement that the stages are clear cut, some people see them as merging into each other.

When children return home they are, observably, often upset. They may regress to an earlier stage of development, they may have nightmares, or refuse to be parted from a parent, or have an obsessive desire to play hospitals. Usually this phase passes within six months but there is some evidence that damage can be very long-lasting indeed.

EVIDENCE FROM RESEARCH

Research in this field is essential. It is all very well erecting elegant, plausible theories; without evidence they do not convince. It is easy to find children who are upset in hospital, but perhaps they are noticed just because they are upset. Possibly there are half a dozen in the same ward who are managing a similar experience with ease. Similarly, it is easy to describe individual children who are disturbed when they come out of hospital; perhaps they were disturbed before they went in. Possibly there have been half a dozen others who have settled back home without a murmur.

A little work has been done on the amount of distress shown by children while they are in-patients. In 1975 M.A. Vinstainer and J.A. Wolfer looked at a number of children undergoing surgery and concluded that all showed some degree of upset, with the greatest being evident in the under six-year-old group.

Most studies concentrate on post-hospital reactions. Conclusions do not all point in the same direction but there is a general trend towards the finding that the majority of children who go into hospital have, up to now, emerged with more indications of behaviour disturbance than they had when they went in.

Although the trend is reasonably consistent there is not total agreement on the proportion of children who are disturbed, nor on the extent of their problems either in terms of severity or duration. This is partly because different samples have been studied, partly because different questions have been asked. Some workers have used pulse beat as an indication of distress, others have asked mothers to provide a report, others have asked mothers to fill in a rating scale.

One common criticism of much of the published work is that it looks at children only for a few months after their hospitalization. One large study which went beyond that was the work of James Douglas. In 1975 he published the results of a follow-up of more than 3,000 individuals, born in Britain in March, 1946, who have been physically and psychologically examined every two years since they were born. Douglas compared hospital admissions with school records, teachers' assessment, and adult work records. The results were startling.

If a child were admitted to hospital only once before he was five, and then for less than a week, there seemed generally to be no effect. But more than once, or more than a week, especially if the child were between twelve months and four years old, and then there was a marked rise in the rate of psychological problems including delinquency, the inability to hold down a job, and even difficulty in learning to read. Only children were more vulnerable than those with brothers or sisters but there did not seem to be any link with a persisting physical condition or with social class. One of the findings was that children going in for an operation seemed much less upset than those in for other treatment. Perhaps this bears out the point already made that it is helpful if a child can understand why he is going in: an operation is at least something with a clearly defined purpose.

Other studies relating to the amount and nature of disturbance after hospitalization are reviewed in *Child Psychiatry: Modern Approaches* by Michael Rutter and Lionel Hersov (1976); and a fuller but less accessible review of the whole topic was carried out by Pamela Harris in 1979.

FACTORS RELATED TO DISTURBANCE

The work reviewed by Rutter and by Harris looked at a number of factors:

The age of the child. It is sometimes said that there is no adverse effect on children below the age of six months and relatively little on those above six years. An examination of several studies does not entirely bear this out, and in any case there remains the possibility that because a baby does not show distress like an older child the disturbance in the younger one may be missed. What is more, the mother of a baby may herself be very upset at having to leave him, and this upset may have long-term adverse effects.

Previous separations. The picture here seems reasonably consistent: previous separations which have been happy are likely to help offset the adverse effects of being in hospital; those which have been traumatic will make hospitalization worse.

Previous disturbance. This is clearer still: there is an indication that the emotional state of the child before he enters hospital is the best single predictor of his subsequent reactions.

Duration of the separation. The general conclusion is as might be expected: the longer the separation, the worse the effect.

Parental feelings about hospitals. Mothers who look back with anxiety to their own hospital experience are less likely to visit their child, although they are more likely to want to stay in with him. They also tend to have children who remain withdrawn while in hospital.

Parents' relationships with their children. Short-term distress has been shown to be less when there is a good pre-hospital relationship; and there is some support for the notion of bonding in findings that a child who has an unsatisfactory relationship does not fret as much as one who had established a clear bond previously.

POSSIBLE BENEFICIAL EFFECTS OF BEING IN HOSPITAL

The children in the Douglas study were in-patients in the 1950s, when hospitals were different places from those we know today. Now we are beginning to learn something about making a stay in hospital not just bearable but positively enjoyable. In America in the 1960s D.T.A. Vernon and colleagues found that about 25 per cent of the pre-school children they studied showed changes that indicated improved behaviour when they got home, and in Britain Pamela Harris also found change in a similar direction. Some of the improvement can be ascribed to better health, but for a proportion of children everywhere home is not all roses.

CHILDREN IN HOSPITAL TODAY – AND TOMORROW

The last section ended with a comment that hospital can be bearable and even enjoyable. This last possibility, that it can be an enjoyable experience, is rarely mentioned in the literature yet is frequently noted by hospital staff. Unfortunately it is harder to carry out research into the good effects of almost anything and it remains a topic on which we cannot draw firm conclusions.

We can, however, be more certain about ways of reducing stress. Much depends on the way the hospital team is able to function. 'Hospital team' usually refers to doctors, nurses, and therapists but in the sense that I mean it the team includes all the hospital staff, including porters and domestic staff, as well as the family and the child himself. In the last analysis we end by talking, quite rightly, about people, not just about theories about people. The rest of this chapter is written with this team emphasis in mind, and in a realization that just as there are good and bad teachers, lawyers, actors, and bus conductors, so there are good and bad doctors, nurses, cleaners, and administrators, often all in the same hospital.

LONG-TERM PREPARATION FOR COMING INTO HOSPITAL

Almost half the children in Britain have been in hospital by the age of seven, yet most medical admissions are emergencies. It is not possible, then, always to give as careful a preparation for hospital as parents might wish. This does not mean that the subject need be ignored altogether. Margaret Stacey and a group of colleagues studied about 650 children who had been in hospital and concluded that those who coped best were those who had received some general preparation in being away from home and in being self-reliant. They were, e.g., used to going on errands and taking messages outside the family.

In a rather more specific way parents can help children develop a sense of perspective about the function of a hospital. It is not just a glamorous place where dramatic operations are carried out to the exclusion of all else, nor is it a place where people go to die. Neither is it a fun place where everyone has a party every day with jelly and ice cream for breakfast. If a child can visit a friend or relative in hospital so much the better, as long as parents are careful to discuss afterwards what he saw: children can easily see a horrific piece of apparatus, or a child in distress, and assume that all hospitals contain nasty tubes and make you cry. Many children like playing hospital games, dressing up to operate on teddy. This is a good time to introduce some positive ideas about hospitals in general – to talk about teddy feeling ill, and then having special treatment, perhaps being rather miserable some of the time when he was in, and in the end coming home to get properly better.

SHORT-TERM PREPARATION OF CHILDREN

If parents do know in advance that a child is to be an in-patient careful preparation can be of great value. Most important is to tell the truth. That sounds a redundant sentence: of course parents will tell the truth. But experience has shown that they are not always as truthful as they might be. Perhaps they will mention hospital and follow up with a comment to the effect that the child will not be hurt. Perhaps they will say the stay will only be for a few days when in fact it may be for several weeks. If the child is hurt, and if the admission is for several weeks, that child's trust will have been broken. If parents do not know full details or if they cannot answer all their child's questions, it is better that they say so, adding that they will try to find out next time they visit the hospital. In this way, if a child has a couple of weeks at least to mull over some thoughts and then ask questions, the panic that sets in when some children come into hospital will be offset. This panic is worst when the parents have actually lied to a child, told him e.g. that he is going to a party or to see his favourite grandparent.

Some parents find books or booklets for children helpful. The National Association for the Welfare of Children in Hospital publish several and have a list of books specially written for children (see address list). I am uncertain about their value. They are, perhaps, better than nothing. Children certainly like them when they are actually in, but often they present hospital as a sunny, happy place where no one cries and no one is hurt. It is not good to make distress and pain a central part of a booklet or comic but I feel that preparation should face up to some facts.

Finally, it must be remembered that not all children will understand why they are going in. For some it will be obvious, for others, though, especially those who are feeling quite well, the whole episode is a mystery. Their ignorance in this area can lead to behaviour which has been noticed in a number of children: they go through an unusually quiet compliant phase for a couple of weeks before the admission. It is almost as though they are saying that they think they are being sent away as a punishment and if they are good perhaps they will not have to go.

One final point: it is always a good idea for parents to promise some kind of present or special treat to a child when he comes home. It need not be very expensive but it does give him something to look forward to.

SHORT-TERM PREPARATION OF PARENTS

Any preparation of children must be preceeded by careful thought about their parents, always keeping in mind two points: a calm parent is likely to have a calm child; parents who can anticipate what will happen will, other things being equal, remain more calm than those who remain in ignorance. (For further reading on these points see the work of E. Gellert, 1956; M. Stacey, 1970; and J. Woodward and D. Jackson, 1968.)

The keynote, as the Platt Report of 1959 noted, is information. Parents should always be told what is to be done to their child, by whom and when. They should be told as much as possible about ward routine, about the best and worst times to telephone the ward, and they should be advised about the most suitable times to ask to see a doctor.

They should also be told something of the admission routine, where they will have to go, what will be asked of them and what will happen. This sequence is often ignored as unimportant, yet it is the first contact that parents and child have together with the in-patient part of a hospital. If in this early stage the parents are hesitant and confused, this will be transmitted to the child and everything will get off to a bad start.

They should, in an ideal world, also have an opportunity before they come in to discuss the admission with the ward sister or a staff nurse. They might then be able to explain that their child has a special nickname that he likes to be called, or that he has his own word for wanting to go to the lavatory. In time the sister will be able to discuss the child's possible emotional reactions to being left, if neither parent is staying with him. Many hospitals have booklets for parents explaining both general and particular routines that a child will encounter. Up to a point they are excellent, but they are twice as good if they are backed up with a discussion beforehand with a member of the ward staff.

ONCE THE CHILD IS IN

Visiting hours remain an area of dispute, in some hospitals, between staff and parents. The views of the Department of Health are clear. In 1975 the Minister of Health stated, 'The case has been proven absolutely . . . any hospital which does not currently allow unrestricted access ought to be seriously questioning why they do not.'

The law, too, is seemingly clearly in support of parents' right of access at any time (see Chapter 8).

Research evidence is also available to back up the Department of Health and the law as it now stands. The work of D.G. Prugh and of Claire Fagin in America has demonstrated that extending visiting hours from once a week to every day is of measurable benefit to children and that allowing parents unlimited access is of even greater benefit, especially to children under five. And yet as late as September 1975 less than 20 per cent of hospital wards for children in this country allowed twenty-four hour visiting. About 16 per cent had less than six hours a day while a smaller number had an incredible ration of less than three hours. The most restricted category was children undergoing ear, nose, and throat surgery: in more than half the wards parents were not allowed to visit their child on the day of his operation. (Information from a survey carried out by the National Association for the Welfare of Children in Hospital.)

It is sometimes difficult to understand why there is such resistance to open access. There is no evidence that cross-infection is increased, nor do parents cause chaos. They are, though, untidy. As M.A. Duncombe, President of the British Association of Paediatric Nurses said in 1966, 'It is an indisputable fact that the happiest children's ward is often also the untidiest.' Miss Duncombe went on to say that there were fears that mothers would disturb a doctor's ward round, yet in her experience a mother's presence usually made examination much easier.

One argument that is still put forward is that children settle more quickly when parents are not there. They are, perhaps quieter, but it is usually the quietness of a stunned child, as was discussed in the first part of this chapter.

Yes, but; while I am convinced both from research and from my experience that open access should be allowed this does not mean that parents ought to spend every minute of the day and night by their child's bedside. There are often other members of the family to consider, the child too may appreciate some time with other children or on his own, and perhaps just as important but rarely acknowledged: being with a child all day can be very boring.

Sometimes there are good reasons within the family why parents cannot visit either as often as they would like or, in a minority of cases, at all. This does not mean that a child needs to lose all contact with home. He can be sent postcards or letters, the former with just a big cross on if he cannot read. He can be telephoned and may, if given paper and stamps before, send letters home.

Some hospitals have a Ward Granny scheme. This idea comes from the Brook General Hospital in London where June Jolly, paediatric nursing officer, introduced what she has called a substitute mum. These ladies, often mothers or grandmothers themselves, act as a good mother would – comforting the child, staying by his bed to read a story, helping to feed or wash him and acting as a buffer between the child and ward staff. As Miss Jolly points out, the Ward Granny is not an answer to all problems; but when one realizes that up to thirty different people may be in contact with a child on any one ward it is likely that the presence of one person consistently, even if that person is not a real mother, will do much for that child's well being. (See *Nursing Times*, 11 April, 1974.)

PLAY

The Ward Granny scheme was designed to operate with one 'Granny' to one child. Another person who is a consistent figure on the ward, although she is shared between many children, is the playworker. Play is so important a subject that it has a separate chapter (Chapter 6). In hospital play is of particular importance to a child for four main reasons.

The first is that it gives him a reminder of the outside world. People who work in institutions, whether hospitals, schools, or whatever, often forget how frightening they can be to outsiders, adults as well as children. By offering a chance to play one gives the child an opportunity to fall back into a routine with which he is both familiar and comfortable.

The second is that it gives children a chance to express emotions that would otherwise stay unsaid. At first the playworker may provide all that is necessary by offering what one has summed up as 'a broad lap and warm arms'. Once some confidence has been achieved, play can begin, perhaps at a younger level than might be expected at first, later with more variation. In play children can be angry: I remember one girl who toured the hospital with me giving vicious pretend injections to everyone we met who said hallo. And they can be sad, enacting scenes of desolation with dolls, or painting lonely figures. The experienced playworker will not pretend to be a psychotherapist, and will not interpret such pictures, but she will comment on them in a way that indicates that she understands that the child himself may be sad and lonely.

Third, there is the opportunity to assimilate new experiences.

By playing hospitals children get to grips with what is happening to them, as though playing through some events gives them mastery over it. I remember visiting a surgical ward and going into the playroom to see a group of eight- to nine-year-olds, all dressed in mask and gown, anaesthetizing a teddy bear. A week or so later I spent an afternoon in an operating theatre and there was nothing to choose between the theatre staff and the children for concentration, care, and application to the job in hand.

Fourth is the opportunity to learn through play. As June Jolly pointed out in her 1969 *Lancet* article: 'The entire purpose of the hospital can be conveyed through play.' An example of specific preparation (for cardiac catheterization) is seen in the work of S. Cassell and M.H. Paul, published in 1967. These workers used puppets to enact the procedure before it actually took place.

In 1976 the Department of Health issued their *Report of the Expert Group on Play in Hospital*. It pointed to a need to help children to play and suggested that one playworker to every eight to ten children be employed, with at least one to every ward and one for every outpatient session. 'Specific provision for play is an essential step to the happy experience of the child in hospital' was the report's conclusion.

For a fuller discussion of play in hospital see the book of that name by Susan Harvey and Ann Hales-Tooke published in 1972.

EDUCATION ON A WARD

Local education authorities have a duty to provide education for children in hospital and for some children the teacher becomes a highly significant figure. Teenagers often worry about missing school work and can be reassured by having a teacher who will go through set books and exercises that have been obtained from the school, so that too much ground is not missed. Most schools are co-operative in sending work in if they are asked, although I have encountered blank refusals.

Teaching is, though, always seen as a secondary consideration: the child is in hospital for medical reasons. Some children play on their knowledge of this and are usually 'not feeling very well' when the teacher comes round. Others, especially those in for repeated admissions, regard the teacher as a familiar friend.

COMMUNICATING WITH CHILDREN

Play is powerful but it is not the only way that children communicate; they talk to each other, may talk to adults when the adult has gained their confidence, and most certainly they listen to adults.

G.F. Vaughan, a London psychiatrist, writing in *The Lancet* in 1957, considered the value of communicating with children just before they had an operation to correct a squint. All the children were about six years old, and forty took part in the study. Twenty were prepared for their operation by having a chance to discuss the procedure on their first day on the ward. Vaughan then visited them on the third and fifth days, encouraging them to talk and ask questions. Each interview took ten to fifteen minutes. Examples of the children's fears expressed during these chats are frightening in so clearly illustrating what is in so many children's minds, usually remaining unsaid. One boy was trying to stay awake all night because his mother had told him he was going to have an operation while he was asleep. When Vaughan compared his twenty children with twenty others who had not had a special opportunity to talk he found, six months later, that the 'prepared' group showed far fewer signs of disturbance than the others. It is not certain that it was the content of these interviews that made all the difference, possibly the simple fact of knowing that someone was taking a personal interest was the crucial point. Whatever the mechanism, the lesson is clear: preparations should not be confined to the time before a child comes into hospital, it should be a continuous process.

THE DAY OF AN OPERATION

If I wanted to choose a single event which contained examples of all the points made in this chapter I would look to an operation day. In outline the routine is as follows. The child is not allowed to eat or drink on the day of the operation – there is usually a 'nil by mouth' sign above his bed or even round his neck. Some time before the actual operation a 'pre-med' is given, most commonly by injection. This makes the child drowsy and also dries up secretions in the mouth and throat, thus avoiding the danger of vomiting or choking on excess saliva while he is semiconscious. Once that has taken effect he is taken to the operating theatre by a porter wearing green. After the operation he may return to his own bed; he may go instead to a recovery room.

Some aspects of this routine vary but on one topic there is more or less general agreement: anxious parents produce anxiety in children. How this belief is acted on varies widely from ward to ward. Some wards actively discourage mothers from being in the hospital on the morning of the operation. Others give every opportunity for parents to be present all the time, even to the extent of being with the child when he is anaesthetized. Is there, then, a 'best' method of handling this episode, and if so, is it somewhere between the two?

My answer to these questions is NO. The reason that there can never be a 'best' method is that any single approach will be suitable only for a number of children, not for all. Indeed, I would go as far as saying that any ward which consistently uses only one way of handling children and parents at this time is behaving insensitively.

Some mothers do stir up their children and are better off away from them, not, though, necessarily away from the hospital altogether. Some mothers can calmly leave their child just after the pre-med has been given, knowing that the worst experience of all for both child and mother, is the apparently callous snatching of a screaming child from his mother's arms. Some mothers know that their child is so dependent on them, perhaps because they cannot talk, that separation should, ideally, take place only when the child is asleep. So, if mothers and children are different, approaches should be as flexible as possible.

Having said that, it is possible to make some general points:

1. Once the pre-med has been given an adult who knows the child should be nearby to give frequent reassurance.

2. The child should always be taken to theatre by someone he knows.

3. A trolley is often unnecessary and sometimes frightening. Many children are small enough to be carried, or they can be wheeled on a trolley sitting up.

4. Preparation for the way the child will feel after the operation is just as important as preparation for what will be done.

5. A child should always see a familiar face when he first comes

round from the operation. Unless there are good reasons to the contrary that face should be a parent's.

6. Whatever is going to be the approach, it is essential that everyone knows about it in advance, and by everyone I mean: the nurses, the doctors, the playworker, the teacher, the domestic staff, the porters, the anaesthetist, the parents, and the child.

GOING HOME

Remarkably little has been written about preparation of children or parents for going home. Yet quite a lot is known about the way children behave once they are home. They often regress, wetting the bed perhaps. They often play hospital games for months on end. Sometimes they are aggressive, especially towards their parents, and sometimes they have nightmares. Usually these symptoms of disturbance pass within six months and up to a point they can be seen as understandable expressions of emotion.

Parents can be helped to cope with such behaviour if they are warned about it, and if they are told that in nine cases out of ten it passes within a few months. Children can be helped if they know when to expect to go home. Some doctors deliberately overestimate the length of stay that is predicted thinking that it will be nice for a child to go home earlier than he expected. This, as a very experienced ward sister told me, is not a good idea, for children need to prepare themselves for going home just as much as they do for coming in. If the date is suddenly changed this can throw preparation awry.

Once home, there can be the promised treat that was mentioned above and, if the child is old enough, there should be ample opportunity for him to talk about his experience and to ask further questions. I heard of one boy who said, in a tone of relief, that he was pleased to be home because he had avoided a terrible operation. His parents were perplexed until he explained that he had heard one nurse say to another that he might have to have his bowels opened.

FINALLY: WHO IS AFRAID?

I have already discussed the point that a quiet child is not necessarily a happy one: he may be stunned. Yet the quiet child and the compliant parent are often seen as ideals. Perhaps we should shift our view and see an expression of anger or sadness as healthy. Perhaps we, the hospital staff, are afraid of emotion? Perhaps we would rather not know very much about other people's feelings at all? If this is the case, then we need to help each other: we are back once again to a team approach to children. As a psychologist I am wary of being seen as preaching the gospel that psychology can meet all emotional problems. Maybe psychology can, but psychologists are as fallible as anyone else. What I do know is that a support group – psychologists, psychiatrists, social workers – can often help children, parents, and staff, providing the approach taken is one of sharing, and providing everyone concerned can admit that there are areas where sharing needs can be of value. The staff member of whatever discipline and of whatever status who can say, 'I don't know what to do with this case' is likely to succeed; the one who is too proud, or afraid, ever to seek help is likely to be of diminished value to the patients.

5   Behaviour problems

As well as worrying about everything else, parents often show great concern about their children's behaviour. With a note of despair in their voice they wonder if their child is unique, if his problems of what they see as naughtiness are related to his physical condition. There is no doubt that there is a rise in behaviour disorders among the children we are concerned with in this book. A study by Michael Rutter and colleagues carried out on the Isle of Wight, published as *Education, Health and Behaviour* in 1970, examined the degree of disturbance among a general population and among children with a physical disability. The findings were unequivocal:

> 'Whatever measure ... was used children with physical disorders showed significantly more disturbance than children in the general population.'

On the other hand there is only rarely a recognizable pattern of behaviour associated with a particular handicap; the increase in disturbance is more general. Relevant patterns of behaviour are discussed for each condition in the second half of this book.

Behaviour at school and at home are often strikingly different, children seeming to be two different people according to where they are. Up to a point this is true, we are all different in our behaviour according to who we are with, unless we are completely insensitive to our surroundings. Classroom control has been described in a number of books specially written for teachers, for example David Galloway's *Case Studies in Classroom Management* (1976) and is outside the scope of this chapter, which is concerned with parents.

CAUSES OF BEHAVIOUR PROBLEMS IN THE SICK AND HANDICAPPED

The causes are almost as many as the children. Some are within the children themselves: those with a neurological impairment, for example, are more vulnerable to stress than those without. It is, therefore, likely that a child with epilepsy will have a lower than average stress threshold.

Some children feel angry at their disease or condition, or frustrated that their body will not do what their brain wants it to. Or they are bewildered by incomprehensible treatments for unnamed and partially understood ailments. Their anger, frustration, and bewilderment has to go somewhere and it usually goes inwards, leading to overcontrolled, withdrawn behaviour, or it goes outwards resulting in aggression and hostility.

Other causes can be found in the way the child reacts to the attitudes of others and the conflicts that can arise when a turning point in his life is reached, for example, when he moves from the safety of his family to the outside world at school age.

All of these interact with the way the child is handled by adults. Behaviour problems are not unique to the sick or handicapped but a physical abnormality seems to bring an extra dimension of difficulty to those who deal with the children, as though normal perceptions of what should be done or what can be done are distorted. The adult does not see a child, he sees a sick child. The first task of anyone attempting to help is to get to grips with this perception.

Parents are frequently told to treat their child as though he were normal. This is advice usually given in vain and, as I said in Chapter 3, it is more realistic to advise that normal bits are treated normally, with allowances being made for the abnormal. Even this is easier said than done and there is always a temptation to give in to a child who is in some way different. In the child's own interest this is a temptation that should be resisted. Look at it from the child's point of view: a parent, or any other adult, who takes trouble to ensure that the child fits comfortably into the world in which he lives is giving an unsaid message: 'I think you are important enough to take trouble over'. The adult who allows the child to do what he likes is giving another message: 'you are different and I am not going to bother myself with you.'

This feeling of difference deep down inside is potentially damaging. It can lead to a child feeling that he can rule everyone, which is worrying because a bit of him will always know that this is not true. It can lead to his longing for the safety that control can bring with it. Either way the effect on the child's behaviour is the same: he pushes the walls to see how far they will go and the further they go the more he pushes and the worse his behaviour gets until at last someone mercifully controls him.

DIFFERENT PROBLEMS, SIMILAR SOLUTIONS

I do not wish to minimize the differences that exist between children, especially when different physical conditions are considered. The anger of one undergoing painful treatment for a chronic illness is different from the anger of a subnormal teenager. The destruction wreaked by an autistic boy who has been left alone in a kitchen is different in origin from that created by a depressed diabetic. Having said that, the basic principles of what is outlined below can be generalized, more or less, to all children, whatever their physical problem.

PARENTAL NEEDS

Some parents ask for help when what they are really seeking is reassurance that their child is not seriously deviant in behaviour and that what they are already doing is causing no further harm. I have found it most helpful to discuss such matters in a parents' group when a wide range of views can be given. When such groups are not available further discussion with parents will often reveal that reassurance rather than advice is really being sought. The safest plan in the early stages of any interview is to listen rather than talk.

Sometimes, though, advice is being sought. Occasionally a simple solution can be found to a simple problem: How can I persuade my daughter to sit on a potty? Buy a musical potty that plays a tune when she performs. But generally it is better to talk around the problem, exploring first the precise nature of the behaviour in question.

BEHAVIOUR MODIFICATION

Once the details of whatever is causing anxiety have been established it may be possible to move straight into an approach, based on theories of the way we learn to behave, known as behaviour modification. As there are books for teachers so there are for parents, for example Hermann Peine and Roy Howarth, *Children and Parents* (1975). The principles of behaviour management are clearly set out in such books. They advise parents to be consistent, to ignore unwanted behaviour, and to find some way of rewarding acceptable behaviour immediately it occurs. Punishment is to be treated with caution and one should observe oneself as well as one's child. There are many occasions when the simple application of these principles is effective; there are others when it is necessary to look more closely at what causes the behaviour in the first place, and when one does that one has to ask what the behaviour means.

THE MEANING OF BEHAVIOUR

A good way of beginning to assess the meaning of behaviour is to consider how it fits into the family's pattern of expectations. I once saw a girl of fourteen who was in trouble with her parents for swearing. She was the couple's oldest child and they had not really begun to think of her as an adolescent. When they shifted their expectations the problem was seen in a different perspective. I saw another child, aged four, who was having terrible temper tantrums, but only with her mother. When the family system was explored it became clear that her mother thought of herself as inadequate in every way. Her daughter was fulfilling family expectations in demonstrating that maternal control was inadequate and her mother was colluding with this.

Anyone wishing to study family dynamics further might read some of the literature on family therapy. A good place to start is A.C. Robin Skynner *One Flesh, Separate Persons* (1976), although I emphatically do not suggest that anyone attempt family therapy without training or supervision.

SUPPORT IN SOLUTIONS

By the time expectations and possible meanings have been explored with a parent a possible solution often appears, with a comment from the mother or father along the lines of, 'I know I should really be doing so and so ... ' Even if parents persist in asserting that they have 'tried everything' it is still worthwhile trying to elicit an idea or two from them. Once a feasible approach has been decided upon help must then be directed towards supporting the parents in the action that they have begun. One way of doing this is to see them at regular and not too spaced out intervals. Another, which can be combined with regular visits, is to ask them to keep a diary. This is often a remarkably successful way of helping parents focus on a topic, enabling them to examine themselves at the same time. The following is an extract from a diary kept by the mother of a four-year-old boy. She had read about behaviour management, she had had long discussions with a social worker about the theory but somehow she had never been able to put the theory into practice. Although the diary did not provide a magic solution it undoubtedly did help her to come to an understanding of what she and her son were doing to each other.

Tuesday 23 January

Mark came back from Barbara (a friend) after lunch. He screamed continuously for twenty minutes. Eventually I threatened him once with being sent to his room and it seemed to work. He quietened down immediately and went and watched TV.

Later when I was on the phone he was playing his guitar and making a terrible row while I was speaking. I threatened three times to put him in his room. After the third time he actually kept quiet.

Conclusion: I have made a couple of threats and I haven't carried out either of them.

Question: How many times should Mark be warned before I take action?

Wednesday 24th January

Whilst playing with Natasha upstairs after lunch he locked the bathroom door and lost the key. I discovered this when I went to get them ready to go out shopping. I was angry and told Mark to find the key. He looked but couldn't find it. I was in a hurry to go out and so after a while I told him that if he didn't find it before we went he wouldn't be allowed to have any sweets while we were out. (Mark has been warned many times about taking keys.) We went shopping. It was very cold out and Mark was very good. In the last shop I bought the kids each a packet of crisps. When we got home I found the key myself in his bedroom door. After tea Mark asked for an ice cream. I said that as he hadn't found the key himself he would have to wait until after supper when we had ours. He waited for us all to eat supper then he had a cornet. When it was all gone he asked for another one. I said no he had had enough. I gave him an empty wafer and when that was eaten he asked for another. We said no. He cried for a bit, but eventually he stopped.

During the afternoon, we were watching TV. Mark kept climbing on me and pulling at me. I told him once not to pull at me but the next minute he had practically pulled me on to the floor. I gave him a smack straight away I was so angry. He cried terribly for a bit, then he stopped.

Conclusion: Mark hasn't been too bad today apart from a couple of incidents, but I haven't exactly carried out my threats to the letter.

Thursday 25th January

While I was baking cakes this afternoon Mark kept banging on the table with his car. I told him to stop but he took no notice. Then I said that if he didn't stop I would take it away from him and he stopped.

The crucial aspect of this diary was the fact that the mother was able to note her successes and failures and could ask for further discussions from a position of at least partial success. Professionals tend to underestimate the extent to which they make parents feel inadequate and a large part of supportive work must be geared to overcoming such feelings. The expert's real skill is developing parents' abilities, not instructing.

SEEKING FURTHER HELP

I am occasionally asked about indications of the need for specialized help with behaviour problems. The answer, like so much of the answer to all questions to do with any child, is 'It all depends'. It depends ultimately on the rate and extent of change that can be achieved without specialized intervention, and on the degree of distress experienced by the child and family. I suggest as a general rule that specialized help be available in the first instance to the person who is helping the parent, rather than always to the parent directly. This person may be a health visitor, social worker, doctor, or teacher. With such backing the relatively inexperienced professional can do a great deal of good; without it he may shy away from doing anything or may plunge in with both feet and create havoc.

6 Play

Play is what, for children, 'makes life real and meaningful'. (Susan Harvey and Ann Hales-Tooke)

Play is just what children do when they want to let off steam.

Play is the way in which children learn to control their bodies.

It is more than just their bodies, they learn to use their minds, too.

Play is really to do with making contact with others.

Psychologically play helps children cope with an uncomfortable world. If they experience something nasty they can play through the event until they feel that they have mastery over it.

It used to be fashionable to try to explain all play with a single theory (see Susanna Millar, *The Psychology of Play* published in 1968) but, as the list above shows, 'play' is such an all-embracing concept that it can be extended to cover almost everything that a child does when he is neither eating nor sleeping. It is more fruitful to try to be precise and consider types of play, so that one speaks of exploratory or symbolic or make-believe play, each with its own characteristics. A recent book compiled with this approach in mind is *Biology of Play* by Barbara Tizard and David Harvey (1977).

PLAY AND DEVELOPMENT

Whatever else it may be, play is a vehicle for child development. Children use it to reach out to the world, both physically and mentally and in so doing they develop skills which enable them subsequently to reach still further. This aspect of play is seen in two types:

Exploratory play. Almost from the moment of birth babies begin to take notice of their environment. They explore at first visually and through exploration come to play with and learn about their world of sight, sound, smell and touch. Later they add movement to their repertoire and as their control over movement expands, so they increase the range of their experience. For a further discussion of this see Helen Bee, *The Developing Child* (1978).

Skilful play. Normally included under this heading are skills related to the use of the body, so there is an overlap with exploratory play. Skills may involve whole body control, like skating or riding a bicycle; or finer movements: drawing, writing, threading, and sewing.

Symbolic play is a precursor to language development. When children play endlessly with toys in imitation of real life, a car or a doll for example, they demonstrate that they have taken a great conceptual step in being able to realize that one object can stand for another. They have acquired the foundation for language, for reading, for mathematics.

Make-believe play starts in childhood and arguably never stops, for in adults it becomes day dreaming. It has particular relevance for play in hospital (see Chapter 4).

PLAY AND TOYS

Commercially produced toys are a useful but by no means essential part of play. On some occasions an old saucepan and a couple of tin plates provide all necessary tools.

PLAY AND THE PHYSICALLY HANDICAPPED CHILD

A common factor affecting all handicapped children is a restriction on play. The immobile child misses out on opportunities to explore; the blind child does not spontaneously reach out to a dangling toy; the Down's Syndrome child will lag in the development of fine skills; most handicapped children have few opportunities to play with the non-handicapped because the latter tend to become impatient with slower, clumsier companions.

What is more, handicapped children experience a longer period of dependence on adults and need more active help to play than their normal peers. Unfortunately some parents fail to realize the importance of play, and with less encouragement from others and fewer opportunities to create play for themselves handicapped children often pass their time in a haze of lethargy. When Sheila Hewett interviewed parents of children with cerebral palsy she found that 11 per cent of the two- to seven-year-olds were reported not to enjoy any activity at all. (See Sheila Hewett, *The Family and the Handicapped Child*, 1967.)

PLAY AND THE MENTALLY HANDICAPPED CHILD

Until the 1960s it was widely believed that mentally handicapped children did not play, they indulged only in mechanical, repetitive activities. Psychological studies have, however, demonstrated not only that they can play but also that doing so is of positive benefit. The outstanding work in this field was the Brooklands Experiment in which Jack Tizard showed that mentally handicapped children could play at a level appropriate to their mental age if they were given opportunities similar to those available to normal children. For an account of this work see Jack Tizard, *Community Services for the Mentally Handicapped* (1964), and for an up-to-date general summary of the field see Michael Craft, *Tredgold's Mental Retardation* (1979).

PLAY, THE HANDICAPPED CHILD, AND PARENTS

'What can we do to help him?' is an invariable question from parents. They can help by joining with their child, playing not just haphazardly (although spontaneious 'fun' play is valuable in itself) but in a planned way, tailored to meet the child's needs. Indeed, to neglect the part that parents and others can take in this area is to lose an opportunity of helping parents to help in a way for which they are uniquely suited. A vague exhortation to 'play with him as much as you can', is not enough. Parents usually need specific guidelines.

First they have to learn to observe their child with developmental sequences in mind. This is not as difficult as it sounds for there are now several excellent aids, some British, some American, to provide a basis for observations (see the end of this chapter for details). Observation means more than plotting on a developmental chart, it means looking carefully in great detail at exactly what a child is doing, what he is not doing and planning the next step that he should be taking.

The second task is to devise means of introducing this next step. To take an example: suppose it has been noted that a boy is able to hold a brick, can let it go but is not building anything. The next stage might seem to be putting one brick on top of another, but further observation may show that this is too difficult a task. So some intermediary stages have to be devised, like putting a brick onto a large surface, say the lid of the brick box, then onto a bigger brick and finally onto a brick of the same size. The observation aids mentioned at the end of this chapter include also some further ideas for activities similar to that just outlined.

The third task is to learn when to start this kind of play and when to stop. There is no rule of thumb on this point, only experience will tell.

Finally, there is more to play than can be found only in a developmental chart. Symbolic and creative play are equally valuable and all children should be given an opportunity to listen to and make music, to paint, to draw, to model, to build. I emphasize that these activities should be offered; the child's own inclinations should always be respected.

THERAPEUTIC PLAY

Most of this chapter has, so far, been focused on handicapped children. The therapeutic value of play extends to all. Examples can be seen during any form of crisis, either a national upheaval or a personal time of acute difficulty. I was a child in London during the Second World War and I can clearly remember the way my friends and I played, with many re-enactments of bombing, killing, and destruction. The sick child will often use his play in the same way, to work through anxieties that he is unable fully to comprehend or to express verbally. A common example is the child who has just returned from a stay in hospital when for day after day the only play that seems to satisfy is 'playing hospitals'.

Psychotherapists may take play of this nature and interpret it. This is not to be recommended to anyone who has had neither training nor experience, but neither should the value of play as a means of communication be ignored. I know a boy of six whose parents divorced. He was reluctant to talk to anyone about his feelings but he constantly made models of birds' nests in plasticine, hiding toy animals deep inside them. His mother did not comment on this directly, but did say, from time to time, how much she, too, missed the old days when the family was all together. Gradually the nest building stopped.

TOY LIBRARIES

There is now a network of toy libraries throughout Britain, forming an excellent starting point for anyone wishing to increase his knowledge in this area. They lend toys and also have a series of publications to introduce the topic of play in a general way. In some cases they offer advice on particular children. Their locations vary, some are in hospitals, some in schools, some in university departments. The address of the main office is given in the address list at the end of this book.

THE HANDICAPPED ADVENTURE PLAYGROUND ASSOCIATION (HAPA)

HAPA runs adventure playgrounds especially for the mentally and physically handicapped, who would be swamped in similar settings for non-handicapped children. Many special schools use them and they are usually open during the school holidays. See the address list for their headquarters' address.

THE HANDICAPPED EDUCATION AND AID RESEARCH UNIT (HEARU)

This has been set up to help anyone concerned teach handicapped children to make their own furniture and toys, using simple equipment. Their address is also given in the list at the end of this book.

BOOKS OR CARD KITS CONTAINING CHECKLISTS
AND SUGGESTIONS FOR ACTIVITIES

Cliff Cunningham and Patricia Sloper, *Helping your Handi-capped Baby* (1978)
Dorothy M. Jeffree and Roy McConkey, *Let Me Speak* (1976)
Dorothy M. Jeffree, Roy McConkey and Simon Hewson, *Let Me Play* (1977)

All three of the above are published in the Human Horizon Series by Souvenir Press.

The Portage Project, obtainable in Britain from the National Foundation for Educational Research and in America from Portage Project, CESA 12, Box 564, Portage, Wisconsin 53901, is similar in concept to the books noted above but much more detailed and more expensive. Anyone interested in carrying out work in this field in depth should, however, consider using it.

7 Sex and sex education

One definition of an expert is someone who always responds, whatever the topic under discussion, 'It is more complicated than you think'. Few other topics discussed in this book are more complicated than the psychology of sex and the handicapped. For the chronically sick the problems are less wide-ranging but nonetheless often still exist. The result of this complexity is that parents, or whoever has day to day care of the child, must themselves take responsibility, for this is an area where they usually have absolute influence during the years up to puberty and even after that their child's attitude to sexual matters will have been critically affected by what is learned earlier.

Faced with the difficulties ('How on earth can I explain *that* to *her*?') some people give up and argue that the sick and handicapped, particularly the latter, cannot or should not have anything to do with sex. In doing so they conform to a pattern of denial that has been prevalent for many years and, until recently, affected all unmarried women. It was not so long ago that girls found themselves in mental hospitals because they had had an illegitimate child. As recently as 1972 Swedish sign language books did not contain a vocabulary of sexual terms. Many reasons, or excuses, are put forward to justify this kind of attitude.

The mentally handicapped will produce hordes of idiot children.

This was a widely held view until it was realized that it just does not happen. In the first place the fertility of the mentally handicapped is lower than average. Janet Mattinson's 1975 study in Britain of marriages between the mentally handicapped revealed that 15 out of her 32 couples were childless and the remaining 17 had 40 children between them (two children had died). These figures are well below the national average for the same age group. Equally interesting was the estimate of the success of the marriages which suggested that 70 per cent were good or moderately good. Only three of the 40 children were retarded, which is in line with other research showing that the average intelligence of children of dull parents is higher than that of their parents. Conversely, that of children of bright parents is lower, see P.E. Vernon, *Intelligence, Heredity and Environment* (1979). In any case, with our current knowledge of contraception there is no longer an automatic assumption that pregnancy will follow sexual activity.

For a fuller discussion of the Mattinson research and other related topics see Michael and Ann Craft, *Sex and the Mentally Handicapped* (1978).

He is really still a baby, I even have to dress him. What need does he have of sex?

Maybe his parents do dress him but this does not mean that he is still a baby. Some parents seem able to cope with the strain of having a sick or handicapped child only by prolonging the child's infancy. Some children go along with this and remain dependent on their parents. But inevitably the child's body will change at puberty. It may still be possible to deny sexual curiosity or other sexually based feelings but one cannot pretend that menstruation has not begun.

He's not likely to live long enough to have sex, he shouldn't be worried about it.

Sadly the first part of this statement is true for some children, but the assumption that follows is not. Not all fatally sick children know that they are going to die, and in any case they have as much need of information about sex as is appropriate to their age and understanding as anyone. We do not, after all, want children to learn about sex only as it affects them, it is equally important that they have a wider understanding in order to appreciate the behaviour of others. If a child with a fatal illness has a sister who is pregnant should he not know what this entails?

He's a paraplegic, in a wheelchair, he must be impotent.

This is not necessarily so, as was stated firmly in the House of Lords recently, by someone in a wheelchair. Even if it is true that a child is impotent or sterile there will still be a need for an explanation of sexual matters, if anything there will be an even greater need for a careful explanation.

He's functioning all right but he's an ugly, misshapen wreck. No one will ever want even to hold hands with him, let alone go to bed.

It is, indeed, very hard to imagine some children arousing affection in others and it is tough to have to come to terms with the fact that marriage is probably out of the question, sexual intercourse is unlikely in the extreme and mild flirtation the most that might be hoped for. It is especially tough when a little girl, severely handicapped, talks of being a mummy when she grows up. It is not made easier by the current view which sees celibacy as unfashionable. But tough though it may be, there is still the need to teach and to counsel.

She may have the body of a fourteen-year-old but her mind is much younger, she won't understand.

Yes she will. She may not understand as much as her non-handicapped sister but if the subject is taught as everything should be to the mentally handicapped, slowly, in small steps with a lot of repetition, then a lot can be learned. It is, admittedly, far from easy but parents can become experts at simplifying. Many parents look back to the time when they thought their child would never ever learn to walk or talk.

The arguments put forward above against discussing sex with children are not, then, convincing. But I feel we must be wary of going to another extreme, of saying that all sick and handicapped children have a right to sex and therefore we must do everything in our power to ensure that they have it. This is the pendulum swinging too far, and in its way it is just as arrogant a view as that which leads to unmarried mothers being locked up. In the last analysis we should first provide enough information to enable children to understand what happens to them and to people around them, and second we should ensure that as far as possible they can choose within the limits imposed by their bodies rather than by someone else's mind. Some specific points arising out of this view are discussed in the second part of this chapter.

SEX EDUCATION

Some schools are very good at including sex in their curriculum easily and comfortably, while others hope vaguely that 'the biology lessons will cover all that'. But no matter how good the school there is likely to be a need to supplement formal teaching. This is so for non-handicapped children as well, and they often fill in what has been missed for themselves with an informal passing on of information to each other. The handicapped child often misses out on this because he does not have the same opportunity to mooch about with his friends, especially after school. In any case he will probably need far more information than his non-handicapped peers, and some aspects should not be left to chance.

Victoria Shennan, in *Help Your Child to Understand Sex*, a pamphlet published by the National Society for Mentally Handicapped Children, emphasizes the point made above about parents being experts on their own children. If they feel that they are not the right people to teach and advise on sex then they should find someone else who is. The responsibility is still in their hands.

Timing is a critical part of all teaching, whatever the subject. Just as we do not try to teach advanced maths to a four-year-old so we should not offer him information in a way appropriate only to someone much older. In conversation children give cues about their interests and knowledge which people who know them well can pick up. If a topic is touched upon and the child's interest is held then it is soon obvious to anyone who knows him that he is probably ready for the subject under discussion. In this way, with a casual remark in the course of everyday conversation, some of the best teaching is carried out. I am, incidentally, wary of the approach which says that one should base one's teaching only on answering the questions that children ask. It is important to answer questions, of course, but some children rarely ask any in the first place.

SOME TOPICS THAT RECUR

Physical changes at puberty

Some children find the knowledge that their body is going to change to be like their parent's comes as a relief. Here, at least, is one way in which they fully resemble healthy, non-handicapped people. For others puberty brings an opposite blow, for even in this they do not function normally. In either case, the key to this phase is preparation well in advance. For girls this means as full an explanation of menstruation as it is thought they need, coupled with instruction and practice at taking care of themselves before their first period. The girl in a wheelchair presents a special problem. Current medical knowledge enables the menses to be suppressed or greatly reduced and this is advocated for some girls. This is not a matter on which general statements can easily be made; a discussion with a medical adviser is essential.

Boys need a warning about the onset of nocturnal emissions, with care that there is no confusion between 'wet dreams' and wetting the bed. (This can happen if the topic is introduced badly.)

Blind children have a whole set of difficulties in the area of physical changes and highlight the need for individual attention for each child. They will not anticipate changes in the same way as sighted children for they will not have seen either their own family or pictures. One blind girl is said to have thought her breasts would develop on her back.

Masturbation

In her book *Entitled to Love* (1976) Wendy Greengross quotes the old story that 90 per cent of boys admit to having masturbated and the other 10 per cent are liars. She returns frequently to the subject in her book citing it as an acceptable substitute for full sexual intercourse. Others have followed this approach and suggest that parents should teach their children to masturbate. A modified view is put by Victoria Shennan:

'Parents may feel that if such a technique has to be taught then probably the need for it is over stressed. Certainly if the young person has already learned that stroking ... the genitals ... produces pleasure, all that is needed is to teach that it is an activity to be conducted in private and for the young person to have sufficient privacy to do what he or she wishes to do in seclusion.'

Physical contact

Most children learn from observation that overt public displays of affection are less appropriate as they get older but some have to be taught this, especially the blind and mentally handicapped.

We must acknowledge, though, that many handicapped children do not have the opportunity to indulge in the teasing and horseplay with the opposite sex that acts as a preliminary to a more serious approach. Apart from showing an understanding of such play when it does occur there is little that adults can do to ameliorate this loss.

Birth control

This is a book about the care of children and it is not anticipated that many will need detailed knowledge of birth control methods. But there is no reason why they should not be introduced as a topic of general interest at some stage well before they are likely to be used. For some children the subject will remain of academic interest, for others, notably mentally handicapped girls, lessons in birth control are likely to be among the most important that they ever have.

Sterilization

For some sterilization seems an obvious solution to avoid constant anxiety on the part of those who are looking after handicapped children. For others, it is clearly not appropriate. The difficulty comes in deciding where to draw the line between the two and no book can answer that kind of question without being sweeping and dogmatic.

Love

So far sex has been discussed as though it could be treated

separately from love and marriage. The distinction has been deliberate for two reasons: one, because some people think it can be treated separately, two, because this, more than anything else discussed in this chapter, is something on which families differ one from another. I argue only against two extremes. It seems to me to be wrong to encourage sexual activity where there is no sense of caring for the other person, but equally wrong to insist that sex should happen only within the confines of love and marriage. The first view is brutal, the second unrealistic.

Counselling

Though left until last this area is, in many ways, the most important. As children get older they need more than instruction, more than an answering service, they need someone who will help them make up their own minds about certain aspects of their lives. This is the time when worries about impotence or not getting married come up, when there is some anxiety that their children might be born like them. Parents may or may not be the best people to help but the number of people who are equipped to deal with such problems is small. The National Marriage Guidance Council, the Family Planning Association, and SPOD, the Committee on Sexual and Personal Relationships of the Disabled (see address list) may be able to help, but there remains a need both for knowledge and skill.

8   The law:
benefits and rights

It sometimes seems that every aspect of life is affected once one has a sick or handicapped child. Legal matters are no exception and it is a surprise to many parents to discover that even making a will becomes a lot more complicated if they hope to leave money or property to someone who is handicapped. In this area, as so often happens in other ways, parents find themselves struggling, using the vocabulary of a battle: 'We must fight the local authority', 'The Law Centre helped us plan our campaign to obtain an attendence allowance', 'If we retreat now we will never win'.

The fundamental subject of this chapter is not medical knowledge, or humanity, or care, or even illness; it is money. If a family has a high income then much of what follows will be irrelevant. In Britain we do not, it is true, have anything like the anxieties over medical bills that occur in countries where there is no free health service but there is still extra expenditure; having a sick or handicapped child is not cheap. The National Association for the Welfare of Children in Hospital recently calculated the cost of family hospital visits: in 1977 it worked out at an average of £3 per hour of travelling time. Having a child in a wheelchair adds measurably to total household expenses (see Philippa Russell's *The Wheelchair Child*, 1978) and, as was discussed in Chapter 2, not only do parents have to spend more, they often earn less when they have a dependent child.

INCOME SUPPLEMENTS

Parents who are living on social security can claim back the cost of visiting a hospital and can often get help in obtaining clothes or having heating bills paid.

Supplementary benefits are the state's 'safety net', a device to make sure that no one has an income that is so low that they cannot live on it. Generally it is intended only for those who would otherwise have very little money, but others, with a dependent child to look after, may be eligible. The extra money given to a family may be used for items like the cost of clothing, or a special diet, heating, or laundry. Anyone aged sixteen or over who is not in fulltime work may qualify, but it has been estimated that over 100,000 people in Britain who could get supplementary benefit never apply. Most of them are elderly who do not realize that the money is available, but there are some younger people in this category. Further information can be had from the Child Poverty Action Group (see address list) or from Social Services offices.

The Family Fund was established by the government but is administered by the Rowntree Trust. It provides financial support for families with a child of under sixteen and is intended to bridge the gap between what is needed and what state run agencies provide. Money is often given for single items like a washing machine or driving lessons and both the degree of the child's disability and the family income are taken into account. For the address of the Family Fund see the address list.

The attendance allowance is tax free and available irrespective of income for adults and children over the age of two who are severely disabled and need a lot of looking after over a period of at least six months. Foster parents can now claim. The aim of the scheme is to make it easier for a disabled person to be given necessary care but once money has been granted it can be spent in any way.

There are two rates. The higher is for those who require attendance by day and night, and the lower for only one of these. To claim one has to fill in, form NI 205, is obtainable from any Social Security office. This all sounds easy and reasonable. Reasonable it may be, easy it seldom is. The invaluable booklet, *Disability Rights Handbook* published by the Disability Alliance, (see address list) devotes exactly as much space to advice on appeals against refusals as it does to explaining what the allowance is in the first place. The problems turn mainly on decisions on what is meant by 'a lot of looking after'. Medical opinions are given by doctors appointed by the attendance allowance board, not by the child's own doctor, and there is often disagreement about the amount of help that is given. Parents are advised to keep a diary, in as much detail as possible, of the child's day and night and to present this with their claim. Advice from the voluntary organization that deals with the child's condition is valuable. It may help to know that 50 per cent of appeals are successful.

The invalid care allowance was started in 1976 and provides for people of working age who cannot work because they have to stay at home to look after a disabled relative. Women on their own caring for a child can claim but not, generally, married women even if they are looking after their husband. This allowance is taxable and can be claimed on form NI 212 obtainable at any Social Services office.

The mobility allowance is what it says, a cash allowance to help people be more mobile. It is taxable but given irrespective of income to help anyone 'unable or virtually unable to walk', children under five not being eligible. The allowance is not enough to buy a car but it offsets some travel costs and can be spent on any form of transport. Form NI 211, obtainable from Social Services offices, should be completed.

Housing grants. Some grants and allowances are discretionary, that is, the local authority may make them available but is not forced to do so. Others are a parent's right providing they meet certain qualifications.

House improvements and adaptations. A child with muscular dystrophy will sooner or later need a bathroom on the ground floor. Many houses have to have ramps built to accommodate a wheel chair or a hoist has to be fitted to a bath. Social Services departments have a statutory duty under the Sick and Disabled Persons' Act to arrange for structural adaptations to be made to a house or flat providing they are satisfied of the need. The act covers owner occupiers as well as Council tenants providing the ratable value of the dwelling is not above a certain amount. Improvement grants are given at the discretion of the local authority and cover minor alterations.

Despite their statutory duty to arrange for adaptations there is an enormous variation from one local authority to another in the amount actually spent. A Greater London survey published in the *Disability Rights Handbook* for 1978 revealed one borough spending £9 per 1,000 people, another spending £448 for the same number. Partly these differences are due to the fact that the local authority is not required to pay for all the adaptations, they usually give a 50 per cent grant, and rent can be raised as a result of the changes.

Families who wish to apply for a grant should do so through their local housing office.

Rent and rate rebates. It may be possible to obtain a rent or rate rebate, i.e. parents pay less of either, if the family includes a disabled child. Leaflets available from the Department of the Environment, e.g. *How to Pay Less Rates*, give further information.

SERVICES WHICH MAY BE AVAILABLE FROM A LOCAL AUTHORITY

Some councils provide a laundry service for the incontinent, or they may help with the buying of a washing machine. Some will help with the installation of a telephone. Enquiries about these and other services should be made at the local Social Services department offices.

The car badge scheme

An orange sticker is available for display in a car window if the car is used for a disabled person, whether a child or adult. This brings some concessions on parking restrictions but does not give immunity from all parking regulations. Information is available from Social Services departments.

Wills

Leaving money or property to a handicapped person is not a simple matter. If both parents die and the recipient of a legacy is cared for by a local authority then that authority can claim from the legacy to pay for the care. In extreme cases this can mean that the person has to leave a Council home until everything is sorted out. It is advisable to seek advice from a solicitor who is experienced in such matters. The legal advice service Network has a sample will which it will send to parents for a small sum (see address list).

Insurance and mortgages

Both of these are matters of great variation. I have known a school to refuse to take a boy on a day trip to France because of insurance difficulties, despite an assurance from his doctor that there was no danger. Other children have had little difficulty in similar circumstances. As more sick children live into adulthood the question of mortgages comes to the fore. There are no general rules on this either, and anyone interested is advised to consult one of the voluntary organizations concerned with their child's condition.

VISITING CHILDREN IN HOSPITAL

In 1959 the Platt Committee on the Welfare of Children in Hospital advised that visiting of children by their parents be unrestricted. Twenty years later many, but not all, paediatric wards have abolished set visiting hours but there is often an assumption by both parents and hospital staff that parents have no legal right to see their child whenever they wish. The law is otherwise:

In the case of *Rogers* v. *Exeter and Mid-Devon Hospitals Management Committee*, 30 November, 1974, Mr Justice Cantley found that whilst the plaintiff was in hospital she remained 'in the custody of' her parents. He continued in his judgment to find that where children in hospital are cared for by the hospital and the doctors this work is carried out 'by the authority and on behalf of the parents who remained in a position to exercise powers of control should they wish to do so'.

Commenting on this judgment, in a letter to *The Times*, the Chairwoman of the National Association for the Welfare of Children in Hospital pointed out that her organization has always supported the notion of parents having free access to their children at all times and that this case appeared to give legal weight to their argument.

WHEN PARENTS WISH TO REMOVE A CHILD FROM HOSPITAL AGAINST MEDICAL ADVICE

If there is reason to believe that the child's 'proper development is being avoidably impaired or neglected or his health is being avoidably impaired or neglected' an application may be made to a magistrate for a place of safety order. Applications are usually made by a local authority or the National Society for the Prevention of Cruelty to Children and the maximum duration of the order is twenty-eight days. At the end of this period it is possible that the local authority will apply for an interim care order, which also has a duration of twenty-eight days at most. If necessary this can be followed by another interim care order, or a care order which can give full parental control of the child to the local authority until the child's eighteenth birthday. For further information on such orders see the book by J. Jackson and colleagues, *Clarke Hall and Morrison's Law relating to Children and Young Persons* (1977).

WHEN TREATMENT CAN DO NO MORE

It is sometimes possible to keep someone alive although they remain permanently unconscious. A life may be prolonged for a week or so, but during this time the child can be in pain or drugged confusion. At times like these parents often wonder about the legal implications of asking that treatment stop. Decisions of this nature are matters for parents and doctors, not lawyers.

LEGAL AID AND ADVICE

Legal aid is available according to income; having a sick or handicapped child is no advantage. Advice may be sought from the Citizens Advice Bureaux, a neighbourhood Law Centre or from Network (see address list). In the first instance it is often advisable to approach one of the voluntary organizations who are likely to have had relevant experience.

Part Two

9   Introduction to
Parts Two and Three

With the exception of Chapter 18 each of the remaining chapters in this book deals with only one condition, their selection having been made to provide a representative cross section of the most serious and/or the most common illnesses or handicaps that occur in childhood. In writing these chapters I have been greatly helped by colleagues from the Hospital for Sick Children who kindly read and commented on early drafts.

The format of each chapter is the same. There is a brief explanation of the medical aspects concerned followed by a discussion of the psychological and educational results of that condition. It is assumed that relevant chapters of Part One will be read as well, since the two halves of the book are complementary.

Part Two consists of conditions which, although serious, are not primarily thought of as life-threatening, while Part Three contains those which carry a greater threat to life. To some extent the choice of grouping is open to question: most children with asthma, for example, do not die from this complaint, and diabetes, if not treated, is fatal. When there was doubt I drew upon an unpublished analysis of deaths occurring in special schools in England and Wales 1974-78, the data for which was obtained from a postal questionnaire which I distributed in 1979.

10 Autism

'She created solitude in the midst of company, silence in the midst of chatter.'

'Our Jane washes brown bread . . . We've taught her that if her hands are dirty she should wash them. So when she gets dirty bread – brown bread – she washes that too.'

DEFINITION

Both the quotations above are from accounts written by mothers and together they sum up many aspects of autism: children are cut off from human contact, they do not develop normal language, they can often be taught to do certain acts but seem able to learn only mechanically, as though they cannot really grasp general rules of behaviour.

The phrase 'many aspects' is crucial. There is no single condition, probably no single cause, no one characteristic type of behaviour, and no certain outcome. The first task for anyone new to the subject is coming to grips with what childhood autism really is. The British psychiatrist Lorna Wing sees two types of impairment: underlying and secondary. Although not all authorities agree with her, I find the distinction helpful.

Underlying impairments include the following:

Language problems. Autistic children have difficulties in understanding what is said to them and about 50 per cent do not develop any spoken language. Those who do are unable to use it flexibly, they echo what is said, they do not use pronouns properly, often referring to themselves as 'you' and speak with a curiously distinctive pitch.

Non-verbal language, gesture, facial expression, vocal intonation, is comprehended poorly if at all.

Problems in making sense of the world. They seem unable to fit what they see and hear into a pattern of experience, they cannot learn what goes with what.

Abnormal responses to sensory experiences. They may seem deaf, yet enjoy music and then suddenly cover their ears at the sound of a stone rattling in a tin box. They may even appear to be blind.

Abnormalities of visual inspection. They look past people rather than at them, they often look out of the corner of their eyes and do not hold another's gaze.

Problems of motor imitation. There are severe limitations in the ability to imitate movements.

Problems of motor control. They flap, jump and grimace and may have an odd posture.

Various other abnormalities include erratic patterns of sleeping, eating and drinking, an absence of dizziness after spinning round and round and a resistance to the effects of sedatives.

Secondary impairments arise from those already mentioned:

Apparent aloofness and indifference to other people, with a seeming use of people as objects. Active physical contact of the rough and tumble variety is often enjoyed but physical comforting is not sought even when the child is hurt.

Resistance to change and an attachment to routines. They may fly into a rage if furniture is moved round or if a regular routine of activity is upset.

Inappropriate emotional reactions. They may laugh and cry for no apparent reason and may ignore real dangers, though they may be fearful of the trivial.

Poverty of imagination. They cannot play imaginatively, show no curiosity, and tend to fasten on parts of an object rather than the whole. They become absorbed in repetitive, stereotyped activities, like opening and shutting a drawer.

Socially immature and difficult behaviour includes running away, sudden screaming, and making embarrassing remarks in public.

Many children, especially those with handicaps to do with hearing or vision, have some of the behaviours described above but they are not autistic. Very few autistic children show all the characteristics in Wing's lists. In order to be classified as autistic, children have to meet certain criteria, sometimes referred to as 'points'. This approach was originally put forward by the American psychiatrist Leo Kanner, who first defined the condition in 1943. The currently accepted criteria in Britain are:

1. An onset before five years of age.
2. The presence of an autistic type failure to develop normal relationships with other people.
3. An abnormality in language development, both verbal and non-verbal.
4. Ritualistic and stereotyped behaviour.

Children who meet these criteria are sometimes referred to as 'classically autistic'. Others, who have some of the behaviours described in Wing's list, may be referred to as 'having autistic features'. It is often very difficult indeed to draw a clear line between the two groups.

THE ONSET OF AUTISM

Autistic children appear to be normal at birth. Within a few months some cause their parents at least to wonder, if not to worry. They may be unusually placid, 'such a good baby, he was', or they may scream for no obvious reason and baffle everyone. One of the first symptoms noted by mothers is the child's failure to put out his arms in preparation for being picked up, another is the absence of normal smiling.

Others, however, develop quite normally, as far as observers can tell, for the first couple of years or so. One of the most classically autistic children I have ever seen said, at the age of two, 'Did mummy put salt in the sea?' He, along with others who fall into a similar pattern, gradually lost his speech and developed many of the features described above.

FREQUENCY

The precise prevalence is uncertain because of the difficulties of diagnosis. The figure normally given is four to five per 10,000, with a ratio of about three boys to every girl.

CAUSES

Early studies showed that parents of autistic children were, more often than would be expected from general population figures, middle-class. They were also noted to be withdrawn, cold, and aloof themselves. Clara Park, whose description of her daughter is quoted first at the beginning of this chapter, describes both herself and her husband as rather shy, bookish people. Such information led to the theory of the 'refrigerated mother'. As a theory it is attractive: all children are autistic in their early days for they all live in terms of themselves alone. If they do not receive adequate nurturing they remain at, or return to, this stage. Attractive though it may be, the theory has failed to stand up when examined critically and Lorna Wing summed up the evidence by saying: 'In general, well controlled studies have failed to show any specific abnormality of personality or of child rearing practices among groups of parents.' Later work has, however, confirmed that there is a preponderance of middle-class parents, a fact not yet explained.

Wing's theory is that autism is caused by the abnormal functioning of a specific part of the brain. This part may be affected by several different conditions. If only that particular part is affected one has a case of classical autism, but if other parts are also damaged then one has autism plus something else, or one may have another condition plus autism. There is some support for this notion in the fact that as many as one sixth of autistic children have a neurological problem in later life. The question of inheritance is always raised, whatever the handicap. Until recently genetics and autism was more a subject of speculation than knowledge but the picture has been changed by evidence from Susan Folstein and Michael Rutter at the Institute of Psychiatry in London. Their study compared identical and non-identical twins and the authors state that genetic factors alone seem to be sufficient to cause autism in some cases. In others brain injury alone may be enough. They conclude that, '... many cases of autism appear to result from a combination of brain damage and an inherited cognitive abnormality.' The inherited abnormality involves language although the precise mode of inheritance remains uncertain.

More than Sympathy

WAYS OF HELPING

1. Parents

A realization that a child may be autistic comes gradually and at first most parents chase red herrings, like delayed development or deafness. (Some parents of mentally handicapped children chase the red herring of autism.) The result is a long period of indecision, similar to that experienced by the parents of children with cystic fibrosis (see Chapter 20). By the time the diagnosis is finally given the parents are sure there is something wrong and they often feel relieved that someone agrees with them.

Apart from the general problems affecting families discussed in Chapter 3 there are some particular difficulties facing those looking after the autistic. One is a result of the apparent normality of the children: autism is, at first, invisible. Passers by then look disapprovingly at this 'naughty' child, behaving so badly in public, or talking in such a silly voice.

A further complication is that autistic children cannot always be left alone, some cannot be left alone for a moment. If they are they can get up to all sorts of activities, some of which are extremely dangerous. I know of a nine-year-old who got into his father's car, let off the brake, and rolled down the drive in front of the house, across the road and into the garden opposite.

Being with any child all day can be boring, tiring, and frustrating, no matter how normal or intelligent he may be. There are, however, continuing rewards from most children for they provide one half of a two-way process. The autistic child, on the other hand, offers a fleeting glance instead of a smile, aloofness instead of enthusiasm, and provides, in my opinion, one of the toughest assignments a parent can have. It is very easy to give in and give up and say that nothing can be done, no one can get through to the mind behind such a fortress. (The title of the book written by Clara Park, the mother referred to above, is *The Siege*.) One of the most important ways of helping parents is by discussing as fully as possible what can be done and how autistic children may change.

2. Management

There is no cure for autism but much can be done to bring some autistic children into something approaching contact with other people. This may be a disappointingly cautious statement to anyone seeking, as so many do, a magic key to unlock the mystery. So far, the only key is the appreciation that autistic children differ one from the other, that enormous efforts have to be put into work with them, and that progress is slow.

Although each child has to be seen as an individual some general points can be made. The first is that the most successful management and teaching techniques are those based on the principles of behaviour modification, i.e. on an analysis of what the child does and how he responds in certain situations. Readers who are interested in following this up with respect to autism could start with *The Siege* and with *For the Love of Ann* by James Copeland, another account of parental management.

The second point is that techniques that have been successful with normal children may be quite inappropriate for the autistic; the adult has to learn how to cope from scratch. An example of this is teaching the use of a spoon. Normal children imitate movement and copy, as well as they can, adult actions. Autistic children do not do this, and have to be guided through movements and actions, rather as one does with a blind child.

The third point is the need to be ready for the unpredictable not only in terms of difficult behaviour but also of progress. Weeks can go by with no discernable change and then suddenly there can be a small flash of improvement, a new skill mastered, a new phrase used.

3. Education

Where an autistic child is educated depends largely on his assumed intelligence and his language ability, the two being related to each other. I say 'assumed intelligence' because measurement in this field is difficult at best and at times near impossible. But if one combines the results of mainly non-verbal tests with a careful consideration of the parents' reports of past and present behaviour then reasonably reliable findings can be obtained.

Over 50 per cent of autistic children have an IQ of below fifty and are generally better suited to schools for the mentally handicapped. This is a sweeping statement; not everyone would agree but it is one that I have found, in practice, to be borne out.

For the more intelligent, especially for the 50 per cent who develop language, there are special schools and units unevenly distributed throughout Britain. (One of the most important decisions of any family with an autistic child is where to live in order to be near a good school.) When teaching methods are compared it seems that the more formal approach, with an emphasis on routine, is the most successful. Some children learn to read and to perform prodigious feats of mental arithmetic. But even the best special school does not pretend to make them normal. One of the most fruitful times to observe any child is when he is at play. Playtime in a school for the autistic is a sharp reminder of just how odd these children are, each playing in his own circumscribed world.

THE COURSE OF AUTISM AND THE OUTLOOK

The most severe and clear-cut behaviour patterns are present between the ages of two and five. After that there is usually some improvement, especially a lessening in withdrawal from contact and the desire for sameness. Children who develop language before the age of five, and maintain their ability, and those with an IQ of about sixty or over have the most optimistic future and respond most to teaching. Sometimes, though, skills are lost as language increases. Many autistic children have special skills, for example, a good memory. One such girl, Nadia, was studied at Nottingham University (Selfe and Newson, 1977). At the age of five she drew horses in an amazingly mature way but as her autism diminished so her drawing reverted to that of a normal child.

The outlook for most, however, is not good. By adolescence about half are in residential care, mainly in hospitals for the mentally handicapped. In adulthood over 90 per cent are unable to lead an independent life and those who do succeed in supporting themselves remain isolated and pedantic in manner. I know of no record of an autistic child subsequently having children. There are many urgent needs in the field of handicap; provision for the adolescent and adult autistic is a need with high priority.

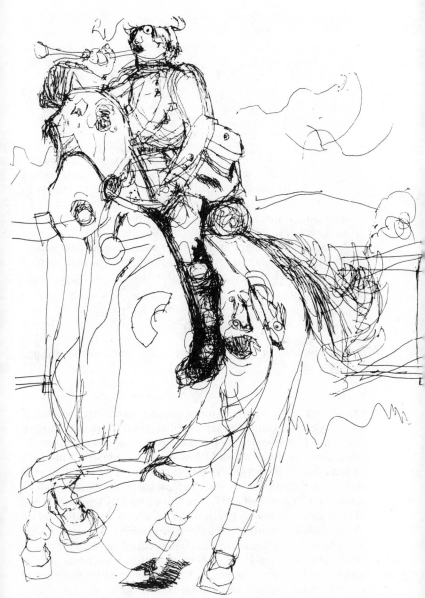

Figure 1 A drawing by 'Nadia' when she was 5 ½ years old

11   Cleft lip and palate

DEFINITION

The word 'cleft' means a split or separation of parts and in this context it refers to a separation of parts that should be together.

A cleft lip (sometimes called a hare lip) is an abnormality in which the outer part of the upper lip is separated from the middle part. If there is a cleft on one side only the adjective used is 'unilateral', if on two it is called 'bilateral'.

A cleft palate is found when tissues which should have grown in towards each other to form the roof of the mouth fail to meet and join. The cleavage thus formed may be in the hard or soft palate.

FREQUENCY

About one child in 700 is born with a cleft lip of palate or both.

CAUSES

Old wives tales about causes abound. An enquiry among mothers carried out in the early 1970s reported that one thought it was due to her having used a sewing machine at a certain time, another blamed having looked at a rabbit and a third invoked internal bleeding. In fact the details of causation are still largely unknown. Heredity is the most important single factor, slightly less than 40 per cent of cleft lip cases and slightly less than 20 per cent of cleft palate only children have a known family history of the condition. In other cases there is probably a genetic link as well, from both parents, leading to a predisposition towards the development of a cleft. What is quite unclear is the nature of the mechanism causing the cleft, the only certainty being that it occurs during the first three months of pregnancy.

From this it follows that the chances of a family which already has a child with a cleft producing another are greatly increased and parents are advised to seek genetic counselling.

TREATMENT

Before surgical intervention became common children had to struggle to survive. Next came a period when they lived but had to endure lifelong problems, especially related to speech. Now the picture is far more optimistic, for modern techniques are such that many children can be helped to lead lives indistinguishable from their ordinary brothers and sisters.

The outstanding characteristic of treatment is team work. Plastic surgeons, dentists, audiologists, speech therapists, and ear, nose, and throat specialists are all involved at some time or another in the long process of remaking and guidance.

The timing of operations varies from child to child and to some extent from surgeon to surgeon. A typical programme is a lip repair at three months, although some surgeons prefer to operate on some children's lip and palate at the same time. Whatever the precise timing, most think it advisable to carry out palate repairs before speech develops.

Further cosmetic operations may be undertaken before a child goes to school but the general pattern is to avoid further surgery until growth has stopped. The provision of a bridge, i.e. the filling in of gaps between teeth, can be considered from the late teens onwards, and in adulthood further cosmetic surgery may be carried out.

This is the overall pattern; some children, for example those with an immobile soft palate, may need surgery at other times and parents should not be worried simply because their child is on a different timetable from another.

PARENTS

Cleft lips are not pretty. They cause intense distress to parents and all who see them, including medical and nursing staff. I have heard of a mother who for days screamed that she could not bear to have the child near her and of a father whose first reaction was a desire to throw the baby out of the window. All the shock of having produced a baby who is not all right, discussed in Chapter 2, is felt at the birth of a cleft child, especially one with a cleft lip.

Immediate anxieties centre round simple survival, with the question, 'Will I be able to look after him?' being paramount. One of the commonly expressed causes of parental anger is related to this anxiety; many mothers tell of not being allowed to see their baby for several days and in some cases not being allowed to feed him for several weeks. Presumably the staff view is that the mother is too weak to cope either with the sight of the child or with the problems of handling. Whatever the motives, the practice of keeping baby and mother separate is likely to produce more harm than it does good.

Later worries are to do with surgical procedures and it is a great help to have 'before and after' photographs of other children available. With such a high prevalence rate in the general population such photographs should be a part of the equipment of every midwife.

FEEDING

> 'They told me I could never breast feed, it was awful.'
> 'They told me I must breast feed, it was awful.'

These two statements sum up early problems: one is never sure how a child will cope. Some can suck quite adequately, and breast or bottle should always be tried first. Some children can suck but have to have extra assistance via an enlarged hole in the teat. One mother I know made several small holes in the teats she used, thus increasing the mild flow sufficiently for her child to use a bottle quite normally.

If neither breast nor bottle is feasible then some form of spoon feeding must be tried. This may involve a bottle with a spoon attached or simply a spoon on its own. Spoon feeding can take a long time, I have heard of one baby who took two and a half hours over a three ounce feed.

One further point on spoons: babies with a cleft lip have to be spoon fed after their lip repair because pressure must not be applied to the stitches, so it is vital in these cases to accustom the child to using a spoon.

Care over positioning is another lesson mothers must learn, the closer to an upright position that can be achieved the better, to avoid food reappearing from the nose.

HEARING AND LANGUAGE

Hearing problems are common during the early years, especially those of an intermittent nature, and can in themselves lead to slow language development. If hearing is normal then much depends on the nature of the cleft, with most difficulty being caused by bilateral or severe unilateral cleft lips, plus palate. A long and mobile soft palate is essential for speech, for without it a child is unable properly to breathe out through the mouth.

Whatever the malformation, advice from a speech therapist is essential, for parents can do much to help their child even before he begins to speak. For them pulling funny faces is more than a game since any tongue and lip movement is to be encouraged, especially those in which the tongue tip is lifted, since this is a great help towards later clarity of speech.

In more general ways parents can help by providing a good example of speech themselves and, perhaps more important of all, by expecting good speech from their child.

THE IMPACT OF FACIAL APPEARANCE

Everyday language reveals the power of the face in influencing people's opinions of the person. We speak of a small chin denoting weakness; thin lips signifying meanness; a large nose, especially if it is red, immediately signals an alcoholic, and so on.

Such is the psychological force of the face that some parents feel pressure to hide their child. An extreme example is the mother who took her baby out in public only after dark. This is an understandable feeling but in the long run it does no one any good. We cannot say that children with a cleft are just like all other children because they are not, but we can treat them normally. This can be done and when it is the evidence shows that children can develop, psychologically, quite normally.

EDUCATION

There is no reason why cleft children should have any special educational treatment, their range of intelligence and attainment is similar to that of normal children. American studies have shown them to be rather more shy in school and rather less ambitious once they have left school but there has been no comparable work done in Britain. Children with clefts plus other anomalies are, however, more likely to be of less than average intelligence. It is unwise to lump all cleft children together as though they were identical.

THE OUTLOOK

With medical and speech therapy services becoming increasingly sophisticated the outlook for this condition continues to improve. There are needs: more money for bridgework, more research into the best time to carry out certain operations, more education of everyone concerned, but the picture in general must be one of optimism.

12 Cerebral palsy

DEFINITION

Cerebral palsy is a disorder of movement and posture beginning in early childhood. It is due to damage or failure in normal development of a part of the brain and is generally assumed to be non-progressive, that is it does not get worse with age.

There is no abnormality in arms or legs in cerebral palsy; the disorder is essentially one of the brain failing to send correct messages to the limbs.

The variation among cerebral palsy children is probably greater than is found in any other condition described in this book. At one extreme is a scarcely detectable problem of hand control; at the other there is a gross difficulty in standing or moving any limbs in a controlled manner. Not only is there such variation as far as movement is concerned, there is a high rate of associated physical problems arising from abnormalities in other parts of the brain and a child with cerebral palsy may, or may not, also be deaf, and mentally or visually handicapped. Indeed, the other handicaps may be more serious, in terms of the child's functioning, than the cerebral palsy.

TYPES OF CEREBRAL PALSY

Spastic. A particular kind of muscle stiffness or rigidity leading to disordered movement. About 75 per cent of cerebral palsy children are spastic, although the word is sometimes wrongly used to cover all forms of the condition. Limbs can be affected as follows:

1. Hemiplegia: both limbs on one side of the body
2. Paraplegia: both legs
3. Diplegia: all four limbs

In fact it is rare to fall into only one of the above categories, when a child is paraplegic, for example, there is often some weakness in the hands as well.

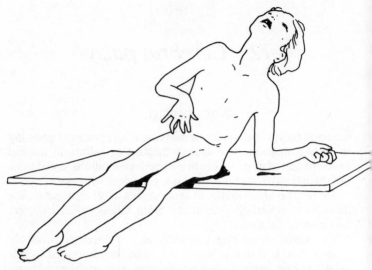

Figure 2   Typical posturing of a child with cerebral palsy, with severe involvement of all four limbs, spasticity, and athetosis mixed.

Athetoid. A condition leading to frequent involuntary movements. About 10 per cent of the group have this type.

Ataxic. More rare than the other two, it is a lack of balance sensation, giving rise to an unsteady gait, similar to that of someone walking on an unsteady ship.

Mixed. With features of two or three of the above types.

FREQUENCY

About one in 600 live births.

CAUSES

The cause of cerebral palsy in individual cases is not always known. A high proportion can be traced to congenital factors, that is those occurring during pregnancy.

Heredity. It is rare that it is inherited; when it *is* the genes in question are usually passed on from both parents.

Prenatal factors. Rhesus incompatibility in the parents, a lack of oxygen to the foetus, rubella, and possibly other diseases in pregnancy have all been implicated.

Perinatal factors (i.e. around the time of birth). A birth injury and/or a difficult birth are often associated with cerebral palsy. Not all difficult births lead to it, though, and often the need to use techniques such as a Caesarian section is the result of an existing abnormality rather than the cause of a subsequent one. (This is not to minimize the importance of good obstetric care.) The rate of cerebral palsy among premature babies is high.

Postnatal factors include a head injury or some other neurological problem. A brain tumour is not the same as cerebral palsy; the effects of the tumour that cause a non-progressive movement disorder become cerebral palsy.

The above list is not meant to be complete, it is included here to give an idea of the range of causes.

TREATMENT

There is no cure, but much can be done to help. Drugs can reduce excitability or involuntary movements but they usually lead to drowsiness which may cause more problems. Surgery is of some value in a small number of cases and is restricted almost entirely to operations on the limbs. Brain surgery has so far played only a limited part.

Central forms of treatment are physiotherapy, speech therapy, and occupational therapy, all of which rely heavily on the help of parents or other adults to supplement work done in clinic or hospital.

Physiotherapy

The physiotherapist advises on physical management with the aim of achieving as much physical independence for the child as possible. This is achieved partly by a concentration on the development of motor skills and partly on the prevention of deformities which are likely to interfere with the performance of motor skills.

There are half a dozen techniques of physiotherapy, all of which claim good results. So far none has been shown to be superior in all ways and in Britain it is common to use ideas from several or all. As each child is different, so he will need an individually tailored programme.

Speech therapy

As many as 75 per cent of children with cerebral palsy have some form of speech or language problem. This varies from a complete absence of speech to a mild disorder of articulation. Children often have weak and badly co-ordinated tongue and lip muscles and this can lead to feeding problems as well as later difficulties with speech.

Occupational therapy

This is concerned with activities of normal life which many parents of non-handicapped children take for granted, since their child will learn much from imitation. Included are feeding, dressing, writing, and fine manipulation. There is also an emphasis, with some children, on the training of visual perception, a point discussed further in the education section below.

In recent years it has been suggested that we should work towards the development of one therapist who can provide all three forms of treatment mentioned above. In some centres there is already much overlapping of role, between physiotherapists and occuational therapists for example. Professional views differ on this; my own is the one which argues for a child having help of the highest quality rather than worrying about the title of the person giving it.

EDUCATION

The measured intelligence of one fifth of children with cerebral palsy is average or above, and some are well above average. But about half are educationally subnormal and many do not match up to the level expected of them in reading and maths even when their level of intelligence is taken into account.

The major causes of such deficits, apart from such factors like time missed from school, seem to be two. The first is poor concentration: these children find it much harder than their normal peers to attend to the work in hand. The second is probably related, and is that of visual perception. Perception here means making sense of what is seen, it does not refer to how well or badly one's eyes work. At an everyday level poor visual perception leads to a boy kicking a ball in the wrong direction in football. At another level it makes games like chess almost impossible and at a more academic level it can give rise to serious problems in reading and spelling and even more serious problems in mathematics. Poor hand control makes writing a big hurdle and it is not surprising that educational problems exist over and above those that would be predicted from a very general intelligence test.

An early question from parents is, 'Will he be able to go to an ordinary school?' This cannot be answered in a general way. Some children are clearly able to cope with all normal demands; some can manage academically but need regular physiotherapy which is available only in a special school; others need the support and understanding that an experienced special school teacher can give. It is an emotive subject in which emotions must not be allowed to reign.

EMOTIONAL ADJUSTMENT

Children whose intelligence is within the normal range have no specific problems of emotional adjustment although, as with all neurologically impaired children, they do have a somewhat higher rate of behaviour problems than is found in the general population.

Those of subnormal intelligence show a considerably raised level of specific problems, overactivity being one of the most common.

It is not clear why neurologically impaired children have these higher rates of behaviour problems. There is no convincing evidence that parental handling is markedly different, and the degree of physical handicap does not seem to be related to behaviour. It is most likely that they are more vulnerable than others to stress and therefore an event which might cause only a minor problem for most children is magnified in effect for them, and becomes intolerable.

FAMILIES

Studies of family adjustment differ in their conclusions, the most cautious view from a consideration of them all being that differences between families of children with cerebral palsy and others have been exaggerated. There is, of course, no doubt that stress is common and the difficulties facing families that are discussed in Chapter 2 are likely to be fully experienced.

THE OUTLOOK

An American study of a group of adults, carried out and presented by C. Swiny in 1975, reported that 14 per cent were married. English work has suggested that only a minority are able to lead socially normal lives once they have left school and when forty-five people were examined in Scotland in the early 1960s about half were employable. These figures are hard to interpret as so much depends on the severity of the handicap and the degree of associated problems. (See D. Pilling's *The Child with Cerebral Palsy*, 1973.)

Any conclusion about the future of children with cerebral palsy must tend to be in the direction of caution. The future is not likely to be rosy, especially for those of low intelligence and little personal independence. As so often occurs in this field, the provision for the school leaver is, sadly, much less good than for those of school age and to pretend otherwise does no one any service.

13 Diabetes

INTRODUCTION

This chapter is concerned only with diabetes mellitus, sometimes called 'sugar diabetes'. There is another form, diabetes insipidus, but this will not be discussed here; whenever diabetes is referred to it is understood to mean diabetes mellitus.

At first glance diabetes seems a mild condition compared to the others described in this book. It can be controlled, children can attend ordinary schools and can lead apparently normal lives. It is rarely fatal and there are no outward and visible signs that a diabetic is different from anyone else.

All this is true but it should not mask the distress and strain that diabetes can bring to a family and to a child. Mild it may seem to a reader, mild it is not to those suffering from it, who have to inject themselves every day, insecure in the knowledge of possible neurological problems, impotence, and loss of sight.

DEFINITION

Diabetes is an inherited condition in which the body is unable to use sugar and starch as energy. It is similar to having a car which has something wrong with the engine so that it cannot use petrol. The equivalent of petrol is glucose, a simple form of sugar.

In normal bodies sugar and starch are both metabolized to produce energy. 'Metabolized' means converted in order to enter certain parts of the body, for example muscles, brain, heart, liver, and kidneys. The metabolism of sugar takes place with the help of the hormone insulin. A hormone is a substance secreted by certain glands, transported to other parts of the body in the blood stream. Food is eaten and sugar and starch from the food turn into glucose which enters the blood stream. A signal is then sent to the pancreas to produce insulin which travels along the blood stream to various sites in the body when it enables the glucose to enter tissues to provide energy. If we eat more than we require most of the excess glucose is stored away in fat. The small amount that remains goes through to the kidneys, which convert blood into urine. There the glucose is extracted so that normal urine is glucose free.

In a diabetic the process breaks down. Sugary, starchy foods are converted into glucose in the normal way but the pancreas fails to produce insulin so the glucose remains in the blood stream until the kidneys are reached. There it cannot be completely extracted because there is too much of it and it enters the urine. Modern knowledge of diabetes dates from the seventeenth century when Thomas Willis used the sweet taste of urine as an indicator of the condition.

Glucose carries water with it, so a symptom of diabetes is the excessive passing of urine. This in turn leads to another symptom: excessive drinking. The body is deprived of the energy normally provided by glucose and so has to use previously stored fat, which leads to a third symptom: excessive eating.

Diabetes is not apparent at birth and may take several years to appear.

FREQUENCY

Diabetes is relatively rare, occurring in about one child in 12,000.

CAUSES

It is known that diabetes is inherited but despite our 4,000-year knowledge of the condition the precise nature of the mechanism of inheritance and the details of the cause are both unknown. What is certain is that no blame can be attached to anyone on either side of the family, and there is no evidence at all that it is caused by eating too many sweets.

TREATMENT

There is no known cure, but the condition can be controlled. The first form of treatment is the injection of insulin to make up for the body failure to produce it naturally. In some late onset forms of the illness tablets can be taken, but children have to be injected every day.

There is, however, more to it than that. The normally functioning body automatically adjusts its insulin production to the amount of glucose taken in but the diabetic has to measure his own glucose level. This entails a simple procedure involving testing the amount of glucose in urine, something which most children learn to do for themselves. It is normally done four times a day, using double voiding, that is the child empties his bladder and then waits for up to thirty minutes and urinates again. It is this fresh urine which is used for testing. If the procedure is difficult or embarrassing for a school age child it is often possible to dispense with the midday test.

Both diet and exercise must be watched. The secret of success with diet is regularity, with the same pattern and balance of food being eaten each day. Diabetics do not have to eat special food ('diabetic chocolate' in shops often gives this misleading impression) nor do they have to eat the same things every day. They do have to have five, regularly balanced meals each day, and children soon become adept at knowing what food equals what. As an example, here are two days' meals taken from a sample menu:

	Monday	*Tuesday*
Breakfast	cereal, milk, sweetener boiled egg brown or white bread marmalade, jam	scrambled egg otherwise as Monday
Snack	cheesecake, chocolate, etc.	as Monday
Lunch	cold meat salad potatoes or bread jelly and ice cream	shepherd's pie vegetables milk pudding diabetic jam
Snack	as before	
Supper	sausages baked beans chips fruit and custard	cheese pudding vegetables lemon whip

Exercise is valuable but it can burn up energy, hence the need to have a snack after half an hour or so. Again an important aim is regularity of exercise.

SIGNS THAT ALL IS NOT WELL

If the ratio between insulin and glucose is wrong then the child will have either too little sugar (hypoglaecaemia) or too much (hyperglaecaemia). **It is essential that those who are responsible for the care of a child know what to look for.**

HYPOGLAECAEMIA usually comes on suddenly. The early signs are:

an unusual lack of concentration
widespread sweating
vagueness and an inability to answer questions
difficulty in reading and possibly in speaking
unusually ready weeping

If hypoglaecaemia is suspected the child should be given sweets or a couple of spoonfuls of sugar in a little water. More solid food should be given once he has begun to recover. Hypoglaecaemia often occurs if a meal is late; a diabetic child should *never* be kept waiting for a meal.

Later stages of hypoglaecaemia are characterized by coma and are rarely reached. If a child does become unconscious medical advice should be sought immediately. **Fluids should never be given to an unconscious child.**

HYPERGLAECAEMIA is usually slow to develop. The signs are:

a dry skin
a sweet or fruity smell on the breath
excessive thirst, hunger or the passing of urine
deep breathing
fatigue

Treatment is the administration of insulin.

It is essential that diabetics wear some identification badge or bracelet at all times.

PSYCHOLOGICAL FACTORS

Regular testing, injection, and diet checking seem straightforward. They can be taught to quite young children, the popular *Rupert and his Friends* booklet (see *Figure 4*) being a help in teaching.

But some children simply hate the routine of testing and

injecting. In adolescence some rebel and refuse to co-operate. Most youngsters use this refusal as a threat rather than actually carrying it out, but I have known extreme cases where hospital admission has been necessary. Other children, not only adolescents, learn that they can use a 'hypo' to get their own way. I heard of one girl who went into a coma in school once a week, just before a lesson she did not like.

A good way to help children overcome some of the psychological problems is to give them a chance to learn about their condition and to share experiences with others of the same age. The British Diabetic Association runs summer camps which are most successful in meeting both these needs. In particular it seems that the opportunity to discuss diabetes in a wide-ranging way is most helpful. So often we tell children as much as we think they should know and then we answer questions. This, as an approach, may not be enough for children may not ask what they really want to know, or they may not know enough to realize what questions they should be asking. Their 'knowledge' may also be incorrect. An example of this last point is the diabetic girl who became pregnant: she had thought that diabetic women were all sterile.

A further result of attendance at a camp or a discussion group is the increased self reliance that has often been noted. This can be a shock to parents, especially to those who started to look after a child when he was too young to be responsible for his own care. The shock can turn to a feeling of resentment and even of loss when parents realize that their child now no longer needs them as he did. As is so often the case, this is one of the areas in work with sick children where forewarning is valuable.

EDUCATION

Although there is not complete agreement on the matter there is little reason to doubt that most diabetic children are of average intelligence and attainment. They do not show unusual patterns of psychological disturbance. With a sympathetic staff they can attend an ordinary school and eat ordinary school food providing the balance of intake is maintained. In some cases it is necessary to have fruit instead of a sweet pudding but this is easily arranged.

Not all schools are sympathetic. Some teachers are frightened

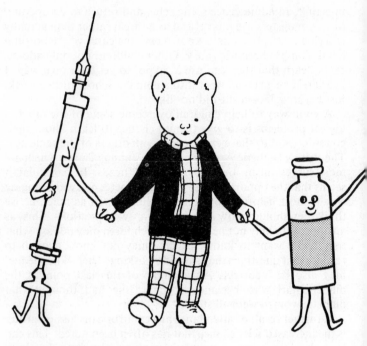

Insulin is Sidney's chum
With coloured jacket around his tum;
Make friends with Insulin
– get his name right
And colour of his coat so bright.

Rupert's just popped up to warn
That Insulin should not be warm.
To keep a smile on Insulin's face
Keep him in a nice cool place.

Figure 3 Illustration from *Rupert and his Friends* .

of diabetes and insist that the child bring his own lunch, sit away from other children, and be banned from school journeys. Others, equally frightened, jump every time a hypo is threatened.

It should go without saying that all teachers are informed of the nature of the condition and of the importance of the treatment. I say 'it should' because it does not always happen: I was once in a school where a new teacher tried to insist on a child eating all his dinner despite the child's protests that he was on a diet. Such incidents are, fortunately, rare and in my experience other children are usually quick to inform new teachers of diet, drugs, and other similar points.

THE OUTLOOK

Diabetes is a life sentence, but it is not a death sentence. With reasonable care a diabetic can live an essentially normal life. There is an increased incidence of infertility among boys but diabetics can learn, work, play, marry, and in many cases have children. The future for a diabetic child is not totally smooth but it is not bleak.

14   Epilepsy

Blindness evokes pity; deafness evokes mockery; leukaemia brings horror; epilepsy is feared. The epileptic child, at least the 'typical' epileptic, seems to be possessed, he is like the man with 'an unclean spirit . . . no man could bind him . . . neither could any man tame him.' (From the *Gospel according to St. Mark*, ch. 5, 2-4)

The vast majority of the 60,000 children of school age with epilepsy in Britain attend ordinary schools. If there is no associated condition their intelligence is likely to be normal. Why, then, is there such fear? To those, like Anne Hackney of Oxford's Park Hospital, who work closely within the subject, the answer is unequivocal: it is because of ignorance.

DEFINITION

A sharp eye might have detected a technical error in the first paragraph of this chapter. I referred to epileptic children, but strictly speaking there is no such thing. Epilepsy is a symptom, like a cough, it is not in itself a disease. We should, therefore, speak of children 'with epilepsy'.

An epileptic fit is a sudden, unusual release of energy in the brain, a kind of electric storm, in which the system goes out of control. Between fits the brain seems to function quite normally.

Some confusion is caused by the words used to describe a fit. All the following mean the same thing: fit, blackout, seizure, convulsion, spell, turn. Some families cannot stomach any of these words and invent their own 'Johnny is having a dream', or 'Mary is off again', are two that I have heard.

TYPES OF EPILEPSY

There are half a dozen types of epilepsy, all of which occur in childhood, the most common being grand and petit mal, that is, 'major' and 'minor'.

Grand mal produces the fit that most people associate with all epilepsy: the patient loses consciousness, goes stiff, and may have difficulty in breathing. He then enters what is known as a clonic phase when there may be a jerking of the muscles. He may also be incontinent during this episode.

Petit mal is much less dramatic and a fit often passes unnoticed. There is a brief lapse of consciousness but the child does not fall down and seems only to switch off for a few moments.

There is no set pattern of frequency of fits, some children have them only at certain times of the day or night, some have three a year, others have three a week.

FREQUENCY

As many as 5 per cent of children have an epileptic fit at some time or another. Of these only about a tenth (one in two hundred) go on to have them sufficiently often to be considered to have epilepsy. Of the 60,000 school children in Britain who are liable to fits only about 600 are so severely affected that they have to attend a school for the epileptic. In a way this is, though, a misleading figure for there are a number of children in other special schools, e.g. for the severely subnormal, who also have fits.

CAUSES

All brains work in the same way, that is we all have electrical activity going on all the time. The difference between the brain liable to epilepsy and the one that is not is one of threshold. Just as some people feel pain more than others because of a difference in threshold so some people are more liable than others to suffer from epilepsy.

What causes threshold levels to be different one from the other is not always clear. In some cases there is another, associated, condition. In others, brain damage has followed an accident, birth injury, or a high fever. There is some suggestion that inherited factors may be involved but the picture is far from clear.

PSYCHOLOGICAL FACTORS

While few people argue that epilepsy is totally psychological in origin some psychological factors are relevant. Stress, for example, can increase the frequency of fits. I know of one boy whose fits decreased quite dramatically once he heard that he could, after all, attend a school that he was keen to go to.

It would not be accurate to say that all children with epilepsy learn to produce a fit in order to get what they want but this has been known, and some children seem even to enjoy the sensation of a fit. I once worked on a ward where a boy had to be restrained from bringing on a fit by staring at the sun and flicking a hand back and forth in front of his eyes.

TREATMENT

There is, for most people, no cure. Surgery is used rarely and drugs form the most common treatment technique. There are about twenty drugs now in use and most fits can be more or less controlled. Unfortunately drugs have side effects and drowsiness may have to be exchanged for a fit.

THE MANAGEMENT OF A FIT

1. *Grand mal.* The general principle is simple: there is no need to do anything except ensure that the child can breathe and is as comfortable as possible. Often this is best achieved by lying him on his side. There is no need to put anything in his mouth or to restrain him. One must be prepared for frothing at the mouth and for incontinence, and one must give him time to recover: he may be normal again within fifteen minutes, he may fall into a deep sleep for an hour.

The above advice applies to isolated fits. In rare cases the child may have prolonged fits, lasting for more than fifteen to twenty minutes, and will be in 'status epilepticus'. *This is a dangerous condition and medical assistance must be sought immediately.*

2. *Petit mal* will pass by the time an adult, or possibly even the child, has realized that it has started.

GENERAL MANAGEMENT AT HOME

Because there is such variation in epilepsy there can be no hard and fast rules about management in general. When in doubt the child's doctor should always be consulted in order to gain advice on absolute limits beyond which it is dangerous to go. The following should be read with this proviso in mind.

Simple safeguards

A child should not be alone for a long period, for example while on a long walk, nor should he be locked away on his own, say in a bathroom or lavatory.

A flickering television screen can induce a fit, so his position in regard to the set should be checked.

A special mattress or pillow may be necessary to avoid suffocation; medical advice should be sought.

Calculated risks

Swimming and cycling are the two activities that cause the most heart searching. They provide a continuing series of questions which can only be answered over time. After all, a three-year-old non-handicapped child is rarely allowed to cycle in the street alone, but by the time he is twelve this may be acceptable. So it is with the epileptic: answers depend partly on the child's age, partly on the nature of his fits, partly on where and with whom the activity will take place.

Overprotection or neglicence

The aim of management should be as far as possible to allow the child to feel normal. As he grows older so he will want to do more and so the temptation to overprotect will increase. One rather melodramatic but telling comment on this is, 'It is better for him to climb a tree and break his leg than not to be allowed to climb and break his heart.' That is fine, but one should make sure that the tree is set in grass, not in concrete.

EDUCATION

The two big questions raised about children's education are

first, how far he may be treated as a non-handicapped child and second, what effects his epilepsy will have on his school work.

To a large extent the first question has been answered in the section above on management in the home. Providing the activity is properly supervised any sport, except shooting, is permissible and there is no need for teachers to be afraid. In my experience other children soon learn to cope with a classmate having a fit and the only drama that is likely to arise will be the result of an adult's feeling of insecurity.

School work is less straightforward. The following statements are both true, although at first they may seem to contradict each other:

1. The range of intelligence of epileptic children is the same as that of the non-handicapped.
2. About one third of all children with epilepsy are mentally retarded.

To reconcile these two statements one must remember that the associated conditions already mentioned are often associated, in their turn, with a degree of mental handicap. This does not alter the fact that some epileptic children are in the very top range of measured intelligence.

The most recent research on children's attainment suggests that about two thirds of them reach the level that would be expected from their intelligence.

Two reasons can be put forward to explain the relative lack of academic success. The first is that all anti-convulsant drugs have some sedative effect. This means not only that children will be a little sleepy in school, the more wily of them will be sleepy when it suits them. I once taught, or tried to, a boy with severe grand mal. After a while I noticed that he was always sleepy in maths lessons, no matter what time of day it was. I learned a lot from him but I am not sure how much he learned from me.

The second reason has to do with the emotional state of the child. There is no such thing as the 'epileptic personality'. In other words, children show a wide range of behaviours just like anyone else. There is, however, a higher than average chance that the epileptic child will be more solitary than most and that he will undervalue himself. This last point, perhaps the most important psychological aspect so far mentioned, is almost certainly the result of the public image of the condition, which is, as was noted at the beginning of this chapter, still medieval. (See Chapter 3 for a fuller discussion of perceptions of handicap.)

THE OUTLOOK

People with epilepsy may marry, have children, drive a car, obtain insurance cover, take out a mortgage and, within reason, follow the occupation of their choice. The crucial word in that sentence is 'may'. There is no certainty on any of these points, but because there is so much variation in people who have fits there should be no automatic closing of doors.

15 Hearing loss

'One of the most desperate of human calamities.'
Samuel Johnson

DEFINITION

There are several ways of classifying hearing loss. One is based on the intensity (loudness) of sound that a person can hear, with loudness being measured in decibels (dB). The following is a rough guide to the interpretation of a decibel level:

20-30	a whisper
60	an ordinary voice at three to four feet
110	a nearby pneumatic drill
120-140	the threshold of pain

A *mild hearing loss* is one in which hearing is not perfect but a whisper can be heard in ideal listening conditions. This is a loss of about 15 to 30 dB.

A *moderate hearing loss* is found when a person has difficulty in interpreting a normal voice at a distance of about three feet, a loss of about 30 to 65 dB.

A *severe loss* is one when a human voice is responded to but cannot be interpreted, this is a loss of about 65 to 95 dB.

Profound deafness occurs when someone has no response to a human voice and little or no response to any sound, a loss of 95 dB or more. Very few children have no hearing at all.

Another way of classifying loss is based on the tone or pitch of sound. Some people can hear deep voices but not those of a higher pitch. The measurement used here is the frequency of sound, expressed in cycles per second or Herz units, abbreviated to Hz. A person who cannot hear high tones will have problems with consonants, one who is unable to hear low tones will have difficulty in distinguishing vowels.

Usually both loudness and pitch are taken into account when

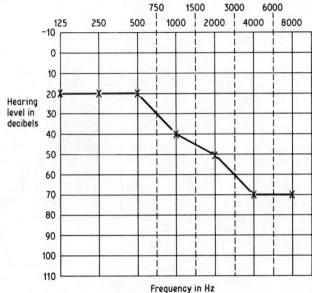

Figure 4 Audiogram

hearing is assessed and are shown on an audiogram, one for each ear.

The child whose audiogram is shown in *Figure 4* has a 20 dB loss up to about 1,000 Hz, which means that he will hear normal conversational speech vowel sounds although he is unlikely to hear someone whispering. There is then a drop to 70 dB by the time the sound reaches 4,000 Hz, indicating that he will hear little of the voiced consonants, like b, g, and m, and nothing of those that are unvoiced, like s, sh, and t.

A third classification is based on the nature rather than the extent of the loss. Sound reaches the brain in several stages. First, in the form of vibrations, it reaches the outer ear. The vibrations pass along the external canal until they reach the ear drum which shakes in response to their impact. On the other side of the drum is the middle ear, about the size of a marble, containing three tiny bones which are connected both to each other and to the drum. They also vibrate. They are connected to the inner ear in which is found the cochlea, a coiled tube

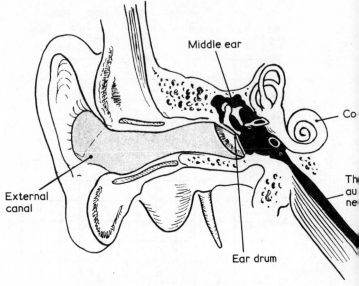

Figure 5   The ear

containing the auditory nerve ends. These ends are stimulated by
a vibratory detector and messages are then carried to the brain
along nerve fibres bunched together making up the auditory
nerve. (See *Figure 5*).
Conductive deafness is that where vibrations are blocked
somewhere along the pathway from the outer ear to the cochlea.
Sensori-neural deafness is due to disorders affecting the cochlea
or auditory nerve.
Mixed deafness occurs when there is both conductive and
sensori-neural loss in the same ear.
Recruitment is found in some cases of sensori-neural deafness.
The child hears loud sounds much better than is predicted from
his ability to hear the quieter range. Thus a shout may be
uncomfortable, especially when a hearing aid is being worn.

FREQUENCY

Because of the differences in classification, and because many children with mild hearing loss attend ordinary schools, it is imposible to give prevalence figures with any certainty.

One survey, published by J.C. Johnson in 1962, produced figures which are similar to several others. Looking at children of school age he found:

0.9 per 1,000 in special schools or units
2   per 1,000 with a marked impairment, not in special education
10 per 1,000 with a considerable impairment which required some supervision
30 per 1,000 with a slight impairment

Putting these findings alongside others it is possible to estimate that about three children per 1,000 have a hearing loss sufficient to constitute a handicap, although it must be emphasized that many authorities would quarrel with this figure, saying that it is a gross underestimate.

THE AGE OF DETECTION OF HEARING LOSS

It is possible to detect a response to sound prenatally and the youngest child I have heard of being assessed was fifteen minutes old. Generally, though, very skilled audiologists can produce a fairly reliable estimate of hearing by about five months of age. As children get older so testing becomes easier and more reliable and at two, three, and four years different techniques can be used with increasing certainty in the results.

Those who work with the deaf are unanimous in seeing a need for early detection, in order that both child and family might have the best possible help at the time when development is at its fastest. In one study of 121 children, published in 1976, Susan Gregory found that over half the parents suspected deafness by the time the child was twelve months old. 40 per cent were diagnosed promptly but for 10 per cent there was a delay of twelve months or more between the time the mother approached someone with a suspicion and final confirmation of her fears.

CAUSES

In a review of the literature on the causes of hearing loss in children, published in 1972, Rosemary Dinnage concluded that in about one third of cases the cause is unknown. A quarter are of genetic origin, and about the same number are due to childhood illnesses. The rest are the result of pre- or perinatal factors, i.e. something occurring before or around the time of birth.

Prenatal causes include maternal German measles (rubella). Perinatal causes include severe jaundice, and complications associated with prematurity, for example, a loss of oxygen to the baby.

ADDITIONAL HANDICAPS

A survey on educational statistics carried out for the Department of Education and Science (1964) found that nearly two thirds of a sample of children in schools for the deaf had at least one additional handicap. In this the deaf are similar to those with other handicaps and generalizations about causes are made that much more complex.

TREATMENT

Many cases of conductive hearing loss can be successfully treated by surgery. Advances in the design of hearing aids and in our understanding of the psychological problems of the deaf child mean that much can be done for them all, especially when early detection is combined with early intervention and when early intervention is sustained throughout the child's school life and into adolescence.

The hearing aid is a sound amplifier which amplifies all sound, not only those of speech. Deaf children vary one from another, and the same hearing aid is not suitable for all. Testing children and the fitting of aids is a skilled task, especially when there are recruitment problems, and the aid must be checked regularly to ensure that it is working properly.

The aid magnifies sound, it does not teach the child to listen. Work has only just begun once a loss has been established and an aid fitted, and most of the work falls on the child himself, and on his parents. It must be remembered that the hearing aid amplifies all background sound; at best it is imperfect.

PSYCHOLOGICAL PROBLEMS

The overall problem is one of communication. In the field of language this is obvious but it is equally pertinent for the baby, for babies communicate, and need to be communicated with, as much if not more than older children. Much is missing from a deaf baby's world. He misses out on his mother cooing at him in return for his babbling (deaf babies make sounds but they do not babble) and he misses out on the reassurance that comes from hearing familiar voices, household sounds and footsteps around him. Isolation begins early.

There is, then, all the more reason for parents in particular to consider other ways of communication, especially with young children. Touching becomes more frequent and meeting a child's eye can be a crucially valuable way of making and maintaining psychological contact. Touch can have drawbacks, though, for deaf children should not be allowed to grow up thinking that a pull or a poke is an acceptable way of attracting attention.

Language is at the centre of it all. A school I visited recently, not in Britain, still has a notice above its main entrance proclaiming the fact that it is an institution for the deaf and dumb. For hundreds of years arguments have raged about the best way to help the deaf overcome their difficulties in both understanding and in speaking, and the arguments continue. There are, though, some points on which most people agree:

1. If possible, children should learn to understand a spoken language and to speak it.
2. Lip reading is inexact.
3. Language teaching must start from the earliest possible moment.
4. Some deaf children are unable to learn either to understand or to speak a spoken language. (Some people disagree with this point; I believe it to be true.)

Lipreading is an aid to understanding but not a substitute for everything else. If one looks in a mirror and says 'big, peg, pig' one can see why one authority has estimated that nine words out of ten have to be guessed. Lipreading alone can lead to a failure in the use of some words. Another look in a mirror, this time at the sentence, 'When is your brithday?' will reveal that 'is' cannot be detected if the question is asked normally. A glance at the written work of deaf children shows very clearly how many such words are missed in everyday conversations.

The main battle, almost a continuing war, has been over the use of oral methods versus signing in teaching the deaf.

Oral methods are those in which children are taught only through speech, or writing, although natural gesturing is not forbidden. The advocates of oral methods say that children should be given an opportunity to communicate with people around them.

Many children, especially those with a partial or moderately severe loss, manage remarkably well in this very difficult task and parents of any deaf child should be aware of ways to help develop language. Various associations for the deaf produce extremely helpful booklets for parents (see address list), and peripatetic teachers are available to visit the homes of deaf children to advise parents and to work directly with the children themselves. For those families who, for whatever reason, do not have the help of a peripatetic teacher there is the correspondence course available from the John Tracey Clinic in Los Angeles (see address list).

In the 1960s an American, R. Orin Cornett, devised a method of supplementing ordinary speech. This method, known as *cued speech* provides additional information to the child by means of eight hand shapes held in four positions close to the mouth. So 'pig', 'peg' and 'big' all have different hand cues accompanying them, although the lip positions are identical.

Some children, it is said, need still more: they should be taught a full sign language. Most deaf children use signs anyway when they are alone, even in schools where signing is forbidden in class, and a system such as the *British Sign System* is seen by its supporters as providing a way for the deaf to learn a language which is, for them, an easier and far more natural one than the oral approach. One authority, commenting on the American Sign Language, concluded, 'Deaf people should take pride in the language they have developed . . . it is capable of wit, drama and poetry . . . 'A simplified version of the British system, called *Makaton* (pronounced Markaton) has been devised recently for use with the mentally handicapped. It is being used more and more widely, and shows promise particularly for the hearing mentally handicapped who have not been able to make very much headway with spoken English.

Others see a need for signing but do not wish to break away completely from spoken language. For them the *Paget-Gorman Sign System* provides an answer and something of a compromise between the two main camps. This system gives a simultaneous representation, by means of signs, of spoken language. It follows conventional grammar, can thus be used to supplement or to replace lipreading as an aid to learning, and adds precision to signing.

Alongside these systems, *finger spelling* (the spelling out of individual letters on the hand) is still in use, both one handed and two, either alone or to supplement signing. (See *Figure 6*)

Total communication is an approach using both signing and aspects of oral methods. The parents of a newly diagnosed child in search of an appropriate approach can be forgiven for thinking that the scene is chaotic. I suspect that it is more healthy than it has been for many years, and that we are moving towards a position where we not only say that deaf children have a range of different needs, we also meet them by using a range of different methods, the choice being determined not by an adult's prejudice but by the needs of the child.

SOME KEY POINTS FOR THOSE WORKING WITH HEARING-IMPAIRED CHILDREN

This section gives an idea of some points that should be borne in mind. Anyone wishing to pursue them further should consult one of the guides written for parents referred to above.

Most children have some residual hearing; it should be used to the full.

Children with intermittent deafness often seem to be naughty when in fact they cannot hear.

The speaker's face should be well illuminated.

A moustache and beard are barriers to lipreading.

If an object is being shown it should be held as near the speaker's mouth as possible.

Speech should be clear and natural, using phrases and sentences which would be used with a hearing child of the same age.

The same word should be used consistently for the same object.

Keeping up a running comentary helps build up language.

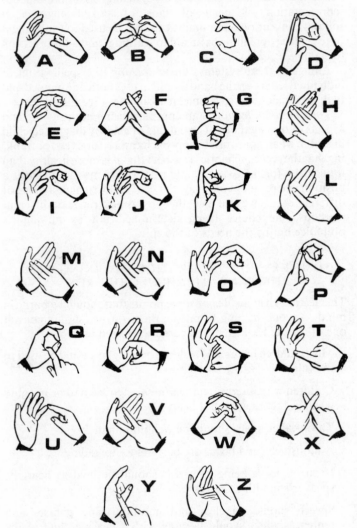

Figure 6 The Standard Manual Alphabet (Finger Spelling)

Children should not have their attention caught with a pull or a poke; they may come to imagine that this is normal behaviour.

A deaf child may point or gesture in some other way to indicate what he wants; he should be responded to with words. So if he points to a fruit bowl, the response may be something like, 'Do you want an apple? Here you are, thank you.'

Children do not learn in a smooth curve. They progress and then stop as though needing a rest for a while.

EMOTIONAL DEVELOPMENT

To say it again: deaf children are different one from the other and generalizations are dangerous. However, research into the emotional development of those with a hearing loss is consistent to a reasonable degree in reporting that they tend to have rather more emotional problems than those who hear well.

Young children seem particularly to suffer from frustration at not being able to make themselves understood. Equally pertinent is the lack of communication the other way, from adult to child. One can say to a hearing child who has just asked for the last piece of cake, 'Sorry, we must wait until five o'clock in case Aunty Mary drops in for tea,' To a deaf child one is tempted to say, 'No'. So deaf children find it hard not only to understand why they have been refused something but also, on some occasions, why they have been punished. It is no surprise that Susan Gregory found far more tantrums among deaf pre-school children than among normal four-year-olds.

A consideration of the adjustment of older children and adolescents points in one direction: they tend to be rather immature and withdrawn, although the rates of overt neurosis and delinquency are no higher than normal. Helen Keller, herself deaf and blind (although not from birth) made a clear point when she said, 'Deafness is a much worse misfortune (than blindness)...it means the loss of the most vital stimulus, the sound of the voice that ... keeps us in the intellectual company of man.'

But comparisons between the deaf and the hearing based on a survey-type approach which do not take the respondent's world into account are of questionable value. The deaf do not inhabit the same world as the hearing and it can be argued that their withdrawal is a withdrawal from the hearing, i.e. it represents a perfectly valid response to demands made on them. The deaf do have problems of adjustment but to go from this fact to the use of words like 'maladjusted' is unwise.

FAMILIES

Many of the points discussed in Chapter 2 affect families with a deaf child but there are some particular problems, some of which have been touched on above. There is the anxiety, in some families, of a long period of uncertainty before a diagnosis is made. Although deaf children do not look any different from the hearing, apart from a hearing aid which may be worn, they sound different, especially when they speak, and particularly when they are severely deaf.

This sounding different, as well as the fact that deaf children do not respond to words as they are expected to, leads some people to assume that the deaf are stupid. It is no accident that 'dummy' is a word in common use.

Parents of an autistic child worry about what he will get up to next. Parents of a child with cystic fibrosis worry about his life expectancy. Parents of a deaf child, especially the young one, worry because of a nagging ignorance of what the child is thinking. Bedtime is notoriously difficult, but is this because the child is having nightmares, feels lonely or is just playing up? At least this is an area where age brings improvement, for most children do learn to communicate with their parents in some form.

EDUCATION

There is no reason to believe that those aspects of intelligence not involving words are affected by hearing loss. Unfortunately for the deaf the educational content of schools today is largely dependent on words, both to explain and to express what one has learned. It is not surprising that hearing loss is associated with difficulties in learning to read and that, in the words of one review, 'There is wide agreement that the educational level of deaf and partially hearing children is severely depressed'.

Where a child will go to school depends partly on what is

available locally and partly on his disability. The choices are: an ordinary school, a special unit attached to an ordinary school with varying degrees of support from specially trained staff, a special school for the partially hearing or the deaf. There are arguments for and against all forms of educational provision. The ordinary school provides a verbal environment stressing normal contacts and standards, but it presents a daunting task to the child who relies partly on lipreading to understand what is going on. The special school or unit brings a degree of segregation, which some would say is a good thing, and offers also experienced staff and a wealth of technological aids to learning.

At least there is a lively debate about special education today, and we have moved far from the view expressed by the Venerable Bede, who wrote in the seventh century that the teaching of a deaf youth to repeat sentences was regarded as a miracle.

THE OUTLOOK

A tiny minority of the deaf go on to higher education and join one of the professions; it can be done, though. For most there is a degree of underemployment, and when at work they tend to be isolated by their handicap. In recent years there has been a justifiable interest in early detection: many authorities see the greatest need now to be in the field of post-school education and vocational guidance.

Against this rather gloomy conclusion can be put the results of studies like that carried out in New York in the 1960s, when deaf adults were found to have only a slightly lowered rate of marriage and generally to remain in steady employment. (see Rosemary Dinnage, *The Handicapped Child: Research Review*, Vol. II, 1972.) Let a man who is both deaf and an otologist have the last word,

'I wasted five to ten years of what should have been the best part of my life as a selfish, depressed and self pitying man . . . I was like an ostrich with my head in the sand trying to conceal something which everyone already knew. It was not until I finally accepted my deafness as an unalterable fact and acquired the determination to overcome my handicap, that I really began to enjoy life again.' (K.M. Day)

16 Mental handicap

DEFINITION

Of all handicapping conditions this is the hardest to define satisfactorily. Essentially, children and adults are classified as mentally retarded according to what they do rather than what they are, and human behaviour is complex in its origin, variable in its manifestation and open to wide interpretation as to its nature. The result is that while there is generally little disagreement about the profoundly handicapped, uncertainty about classification increases the closer the child's behaviour is to the normal.

From the earliest times, and in this case the earliest times in England refers to the thirteenth century, there have been attempts at defining categories of mental handicap. In the reign of Edward I a distinction was made between the 'born fool' and the 'lunatic'. By the sixteenth century the word 'idiot' was being used to describe anyone subnormal, or ignorant and uneducated and by the nineteenth century terminology had become refined to the extent of using three categories: idiot (the lowest), imbecile, and feeble-minded or moron.

Modern distinctions date from the 1944 Education Act when educationally subnormal children were defined as (a) those of limited ability and (b) those retarded by 'other conditions' (such as irregular attendance and ill health,) who were educationally retarded by more than 20 per cent for their age. Below this group were the 'ineducable' known as the severely subnormal (SSN) who were to be cared for by health rather than educational authorities.

In Britain this position changed in 1971 following the 1970 Education (Handicapped Children) Act and all children are now seen as likely to benefit from education. The categories formerly called ESN and ineducable have been replaced by ESN(M) and ESN(S), with M standing for moderate and S for severe.

In 1968 the World Health Organisation suggested a more complex refinement of categories, which is given on page 124. In many ways I find this classification more helpful than the British crude distinctions, but this is a problem that has been with us for some 700 years and it seems likely that we shall be searching both for suitable words and suitable classification systems for some time to come.

The most commonly used measurement technique in this field is the intelligence test which gives a result for each person expressed as an IQ (Intelligence Quotient). Most tests have an IQ of 100 as average, with 68 per cent of any normal population scoring between 85 and 115 and about 2.3 per cent getting scores of below 70. The use of the concept of 'mental age' is, in my opinion, of uncertain value. A twelve-year-old with a so-called mental age of five years is quite different from a three-year-old with a mental age of five.

The ready assumption that anyone with an IQ of 70 or below should be regarded as ESN has recently been heavily criticized on several accounts: tests look at only a sample of what the person can do, they do not measure qualities like persistence or curiosity. Results reflect what a child has learned rather than what he may learn given optional conditions. And no test has yet been devised to enable us to consider a child independently of his cultural background. Further criticisms involve the possibility that both the place of testing and the personality of the tester can affect scores. I do not go along with the argument that all intelligence tests should be abolished but I do think there is much support for criticisms that have been made, and I welcome the swing towards looking at as many factors as possible when trying to come to what often amounts to an administrative decision about a child. Today we should, if possible, look at the IQ, a detailed developmental history, a medical report, teachers' comments, and opinions from parents before we begin to label a child as subnormal. Many education authorities do not accept even this evidence and have set up assessment centres where children can be observed over several weeks or even months before a decision on where he should go is made.

So, with a degree of caution about the validity of the IQ, we can consider what definitions actually mean. The following table is based on an amalgamation of several sources and draws quite heavily on reports from the American President's Panel on Mental Retardation.

As has already been said, classification is no easy matter and the table below is intended to give an indication of a person's performance, it is emphatically not meant to represent clear, cut and dried, separate groups.

Classifications of subnormality

W.H.O. terminology	British terminology	Years	
Profound IQ 0-20	ESN (S)	0-5:	Gross retardation, needing nursing care.
		6-21:	Obvious delays in all areas; few learn to walk or to have simple speech.
		Adult:	Incapable of self maintenance.
Severe IQ 20-30	ESN (S)	0-5:	Marked delay in all development.
		6-21:	Some understanding of speech;
		Adult:	Can perform simple daily tasks but needs constant supervision.
Moderate IQ 30-50	ESN (S)	0-5:	Noticeable delay in motor and language development.
		6-21:	Can learn simple communication skills and safety habits; may read but with little understanding, likely to remain very childish in behaviour and interests.
		Adult:	Needs supervision to carry out simple tasks; can travel alone in familiar areas; usually incapable of self maintenance.
Mild IQ 50-75	ESN (M)	0-5:	Often not noticed as retarded but probably slow to walk and more probably slow to talk.
		6-21:	Can acquire practical skills and may become literate.

Adult: Can usually maintain self, although guidance and support may be needed especially over financial matters.

FREQUENCY

If we worked only on IQ figures we could say that about twenty-three children in every 1,000 are subnormal. But we do not, and to some extent prevalence figures reflect the extent of provision: when we have more places in special schools or units we have more ESN pupils. A general figure is six to seven in every 10,000 ESN(S), while the total population of the subnormal, from profound to borderline, is about one in every 100 children.

CAUSES

A survey of a group of ESN(S) children, published in 1963, revealed that the cause of this handicap was unknown in two thirds of the cases studied. More recently the National Society for Mentally Handicapped Children concluded that the cause of subnormality is 'still largely a mystery'. (See A.M. Clarke and A.D.B. Clarke *Readings from Mental Deficiency*, 1978.)

ESN(S) children are nearly always assumed to have some organic disease or pathology which underlies their difficulties. Often their retardation is associated with a known syndrome or with another handicap; at least 300 other conditions are known to be linked with a degree of subnormality. But in turn the cause of the overall syndrome may also be unknown.

ESN(M) children present a different picture. Some can be explained as the result of normal genetic variation: as a proportion of children are born bright, so a proportion are born well below average. (Not all psychologists agree with this view but it makes sense to me.) Organic defects, that is structural weaknesses in the brain, also play their part in this group but, to a far greater extent than is so with the ESN(S), factors to do with upbringing are implicated. The argument is that some children are either subnormal or so labelled (and the two may not mean the same thing) because their upbringing has either been deficient or because it has been drastically different from that which most children in a certain society enjoy. An extreme case I came across was that of a mother of a four-year-old non-speaking boy who told me that she had tried talking to him when he was a year old but he had not understood so she had given up. Less extreme cases are those families where there are no toys and play is discouraged, where conversation is minimal and where no one ever reads. Often environmental influences interact with others to make matters worse and it is far from easy to disentangle them.

Known causes

These fall into three main groups:

1. A specified genetic origin can be related to harmful genes, inherited from either parent, or to aberrant chromosomes. Chromosomes provide the programme for development and if there is a fault in their structure then development will be affected. The most common example is Down's Syndrome, the largest single condition in the field of mental handicap, which has an incidence of about one in 700 births and may account for as many as a quarter of all severely handicapped children.

2. Environmental factors of an organic nature can be subdivided into three groups.

Prenatal include rubella (German measles) contracted by the mother during early pregnancy, and congenital syphilis.

Perinatal (around the time of birth) include a lack of oxygen to the baby, or birth complications leading to injury.

Postnatal include a very wide range of illnesses and events. A child chewing a window frame painted in lead paint can become poisoned; meningitis or whooping cough can lead to retardation, as can a severe blow to the head, for example in a road accident.

3. Environmental factors of a non-organic nature include those aspects of upbringing which have been mentioned already. They are especially noticeable in children who have been brought up in institutions, although it must be noted that being in an institution is not in itself a guarantee that a child will be retarded. It is not as simple as that.

Neither is it correct to assume that early experience is

everything. It is undoubtedly important but the idea that all intelligence is fixed, if not at birth then within the first five years of life, is now seen to be an assumption without foundation. (On this topic see, for example, essays in *Early Experience: Myth and Evidence*, edited by A.M. and A.D.B. Clarke.)

'It is not as simple as that' is really a refrain for this section. It is hard for parents to hear that no one can necessarily give a reason for their child's slow development; it is almost as hard to have to say this to parents.

MANAGEMENT

Next after 'why?' and 'what is the outlook?' comes the question 'what can I do?' This is an area in which there have been exciting developments in the last few years and in which work continues. The emphasis of research has been partly in seeing what retarded children can, in fact, learn and, latterly, on how far parents can act as partners in helping this learning take place. No single profession has the answer to all problems and much depends on the availability of a range of specialists, plus their ability to work co-operatively.

The starting point is always where the child is at. What can he do, what can't he do, what can we expect next? We know that the severely retarded have, by definition, brains that do not develop as fast or as fully as a normal child's does, but we need to consider in more detail what this means in practice. The retarded child goes through developmental stages in the same sequence as the normal but does so much more slowly and in almost all cases comes to a halt before the final stages have been reached.

In looking at children in detail it helps to do so in two different ways. The first is a general one and relates to areas of lag or deficiency. For example, the retarded are often found to have weaknesses in some or all of the following:

1. Abstract thinking: they stick to concrete ideas and find symbolic reasoning impossible to cope with.
2. Attention: it is often very hard to get them to concentrate on a particular topic and to attend to the essential task in hand.
3. Incoming sensory information: they may hear and see perfectly well but not be able to make sense or use of what comes of them.

4. Memory, both visual and auditory. Sometimes, though, they have what seems, by comparison to their other skills, to be a good memory. For example, they remember what they have seen on television. This can give a misleading impression of intelligence.

5. Incidental learning: normal children pick up an enormous amount as they go along; they seem to absorb information like a sponge and they can often work something out for themselves. Some even teach themselves to read. But the retarded child needs much more conscious teaching.

The second way to look at a child is to make detailed observations of what he is able to do and then to play how to help him. Ideally this should be done by a parent working in conjunction with one or more professionals, but parents alone can do much, especially if they have someone else with whom to discuss their observations. Several books in the Human Horizon series (see Chapter 5) have been written for parents to help them observe their children systematically.

Once a careful observation has been made work can start to encourage the child to reach the next stage. This sounds easy on paper. Experience has shown that it can be done with success, but it is not as easy as it may sound. Parents need encouragement to continue: they may try something for a week or so and then give up, not realizing that the retarded child needs far more repetition, far more careful structuring of what is done and far more breaking an activity down into small steps than is required for a normal child. Parents also need encouragement, at times, to stop: going too fast in, say, language development, can lead only to a child clamming up and saying nothing. Fortunately needs in this area are now recognized and in many places are being met. Hampshire, for example, has a system based on the American Portage Project in which parents of mentally handicapped pre-school children are visited every week, a careful monitoring of their child's progress being part of the scheme. The Hester Adrian Centre in Manchester has pioneered work with parents and there is a steadily growing body of knowledge in this field.

LANGUAGE

Although language is only one part of a child's development it is so central to every other aspect of behaviour that it deserves a separate section. Language is more than speech; it encompasses comprehension as well as expression and is invariably slow to develop in retarded children. The following points should be kept in mind by anyone working with a retarded child:

His comprehension may be much greater than his powers of expression but this is not always the case.

He may know what he wants to express but poor articulation can get in the way of his saying it properly.

He may not notice that others do not properly understand and so may maintain faulty habits.

His memory is likely to be poor so he will not easily learn certain word patterns that other children grasp quickly. For example, he may continue to say 'boy good' instead of 'good boy'.

He may not pick up non-verbal cues, facial expression, for example, or tone of voice.

The greater his retardation the greater the delay, especially of sentence length and complexity. Language tends to remain at a primitive level.

With age, language delay becomes a deviance. At first it is just delayed but the lag often gets greater. In Down's Syndrome this is especially likely, and by maturity development has stopped at a stage where the lag constitutes not just a delay but an actual difference.

Some children are helped by a sign system used in conjunction with speech. The Makaton System has been particularly successful in this way (see Chapter 16).

For others the system of pictorial symbols on a board, known as Bliss Symbols, is more useful. This requires only that children point to a symbol or series of symbols, underneath each of which is written the meaning so that anyone may understand and reply.

Delayed language is not in itself an indication of sub-normality. The child may be deaf or suffer from a specific language delay requiring specialized help. The Association for All Speech-Impaired Children may be able to help in such cases (see address list).

EMOTIONAL DEVELOPMENT

The emotional needs of the subnormal are no different from those of anyone else. They need security, a sense of being accepted by others, a feeling of self esteem and of independence within their own limits. The first is often provided in abundance at the expense of independence. Children can easily find their self esteem dented, especially if they remain the 'dummy' in an ordinary school. Their physical and emotional development may not be in step, with the result that one is faced with what seems to be a big baby. At times the childlike spontaneity and lack of inhibition of the subnormal can lead to embarrassment in public, for these children say what they mean no matter who is around to hear them. Parents and teachers need an X-ray eye at times: they have to be able to look through the physique to the mind behind it.

BEHAVIOUR PROBLEMS

The rate of behaviour problems among the subnormal is higher than is found in the general population. In this context I am referring to problems of hyperactivity, of tantrums, of mannerisms which include rocking and hand flapping and, in extreme, distressing cases, of self mutilation. As there is no single cause of subnormality so there is no single cause of behaviour problems but there are some general points to consider.

The first question always to ask when any behaviour is causing distress is, why is it happening? What does it do for the person who is doing it? With the severely and profoundly mentally handicapped this is far from easy to unravel, for there may be a cause which is not readily apparent, like toothache, which the child feels but is unable to talk about.

Often, though, it is possible to come to some conclusions about the results of the child's behaviour from a straightforward observation of what happens when he does something. Is he rewarded by extra attention? Does he then repeat the act? If so, a change in the response pattern is required. This is discussed more fully in Chapter 5.

A thread that runs through much behaviour is communication. Much so-called difficult behaviour is an imperfect substitute for communication by more conventional means, and the single most effective technique for overcoming problems is the development of a way of exchanging thoughts with a child. I am thinking now of a boy I knew, severely handicapped, hyperactive, very noisy, very aggressive. After many months' hard work his parents taught him that clapping was a sign of approval and immediately his problems lessened appreciably because there was at last a way available for the parents to communicate and to shape what he did. He did not, incidentally, become calm and quiet overnight, but he was easier to manage. Another child, a twelve-year-old girl unable to speak, presented difficulties to her teachers for years. Then she learned a few Makaton signs and suddenly her life was transformed into one in which she had contact with others. Isolation is terrible, whatever your mental age.

THE LAW

General legal topics are discussed in Chapter 8. Parents of the subnormal, though, need to have more than a general knowledge, they should be thoroughly acquainted with a number of particular points.

One example is what to do and say if a subnormal person commits an offence. From time to time this happens. The crucial question is whether the person concerned understood what he was doing. If he is an adult (and the age of minority stops at eighteen for everyone) he may find himself in prison for something he does not comprehend. If, on the other hand, a defence of unfit to plead is put forward he may find himself in a 'Special Hospital', and designated a danger to society.

At times like this expert legal advice is essential and help should be sought before statements are made. The National Society for Mentally Handicapped children and the National Association for Mental Health can give further advice on how to prepare for these and other eventualities.

EDUCATION

The possibilities are: an ordinary school, a special class or unit within an ordinary school, a special school for the ESN(M) or (S) or an institution, which normally means a mental hospital. A minority of children are taught outside the state system, for example in Steiner Schools, many of which do a first rate job.

Decisions about school at the age of five are often the most difficult of all. This is the time when the child is presented to the world, when he has to sink or swim. Careful pre-school assessment, based on repeated observations rather than a quick one-off visit, can often enable wise decisions to be made and provision to be organized well in advance. Once a child is in school there may be pressure on the parents to consider a transfer to what is usually in their eyes an inferior place. The hardest task at times like this is disentangling emotional and educational needs from social stigma. I put emotional needs first because there is virtually no evidence that subnormal children do any better academically in special schools than they do in ordinary education. But there is some evidence, for example from the comparative work of the psychologist Len Green, that they are happier.

In theory, transfer back to mainstream education is possible and I have known it happen. It is rare, though, partly because teachers in special schools often do not feel that the children can cope in an ordinary school, partly because parents are frequently very pleased with their child's education, and partly because authorities have, in the last ten years or so, become far more sophisticated in their assessment techniques.

Deciding on school placement sounds as if it should be straightforward, and when severely handicapped children are concerned it usually is. The problems arise with the ESN(M), especially those on the borderline between special and ordinary school, for many parents resist and resist again any suggestion of a transfer. They insist that the child is normal, he just can't understand that particular teacher/psychologist/paediatrician; or he is a bit off colour every time he is tested or observed; or he is lazy. The mechanism behind such thoughts is easy to interpret, there remains a lingering hope that the child is, after all, normal.

Anyone reading the last few paragraphs may think that I am carrying on a campaign for special schools, against parents. On the whole, if I am to declare a preference, I think special schools for the subnormal do well and provide much. But I have known bad schools, I have known children score consistently low on intelligence tests and yet hold their own in ordinary schools, I have known children transfer back from a special school to a comprehensive in the teeth of opposition from the special school head, and make a success of it. One lesson I have learned is never to make a hasty judgement.

INSTITUTIONS

This is not a book about institutional care. Nevertheless, the topic is relevant for those looking after the retarded at home, because of the pressures for and against institutional life that can be brought to bear. A couple of generations ago, it was not uncommon to hear parents say that the only advice given by any professional was, 'Put him away, mother, and forget all about him'. Then the pendulum began to swing and today official policy is to reduce as far as possible the number of mentally handicapped people in large institutions, with a corresponding emphasis now both on helping parents keep a child at home and on the setting up of small hostels in the community.

It is likely that most parents do want to keep their children with them as long as possible. This was the clear conclusion of a study of 250 severely retarded children's families published by Jack Tizard and J.G. Grad in 1961. But some parents cannot cope. Short term care, for a week or so, is a great help but there remain some situations where the constant care that is required can no longer be provided. Parents are then in a dilemma for they may feel guilty at flying in the face of received opinion. As so often is the case, one cannot make sweeping generalizations about this problem; each case has its own arguments.

THE FAMILY

General family considerations are discussed in Chapter 2. There is one question affecting nearly all families of the retarded, especially those in the ESN(S) group and that is, 'What will happen when we can no longer look after him?' Knowledge about constraints on a will bequeathing money or property to a mentally handicapped person is essential (see Chapter 8). One solution is to set up a Trust Fund, advice on which can be had from the National Society for Mentally Handicapped Children. The National Society also administers the Trusteeship Scheme, by which parents can esure that their child will have a specially appointed visitor who will keep in regular contact with him when they are no longer here to do this themselves. Total parental care can never be replaced but this scheme goes a little way towards mitigating the loss of an adult child's parents.

THE OUTLOOK

The outlook for the profoundly handicapped child is one of continuing care by others; there is no possibility that he will gain independence.

The outlook for the child near the borderline of ESN(M) and normal gets better the older he becomes, for as school is left behind so academic demands are no longer made on him and he can, at least in a time of reasonable employment, find and hold a job. Certainly marriage and parenthood are both possible and probable. There seems, indeed, to be what has been referred to as 'a self righting tendency which appears to move children in the direction of normality in the face of pressure towards deviation' (Sameroff and Chandler, 1975).

Between these two extremes lies the whole range of children and the whole range of possibilities. Much depends on the society in which the person moves. In some circles, a mildly subnormal man or woman will pass unnoticed; in others they are an embarrassment to everyone. With that warning in mind, we can turn with some optimism to the conclusion of an American 1972 review of what is known about adults, written by H.V. Cobb. It was, 'The most consistent and outstanding finding . . . is the high proportion of the adult retarded who achieve satisfactory adjustments, by whatever criteria one employed.'

17   Visual loss

Many people think that blindness is the ultimate in handicaps. To call someone a spastic is a term of abuse in some circles. I have heard children use the word in a playground when someone drops a catch. The word leukaemia is frightening; mental handicap is somehow not quite nice, but blindness inevitably evokes pity.

This extremity of emotion gets in the way both of helping and understanding the visually handicapped. In the first place the pity is often misplaced and, quite rightly, resented by the handicapped. In the second the picture of total darkness conjured up by the word blindness is accurate for only about 10 per cent of those who are registered blind: the other 90 per cent all have some remaining sight. As a senior member of one of the leading charities for the blind put it to me: 'Our greatest enemy is the person who talks to parents about what children cannot see; we want to emphasize the extent to which most of them can use their eyes.'

DEFINITIONS OF VISUAL HANDICAP

There is no single, generally accepted, definition of visual handicap. Essentially, as far as children are concerned, it is a matter for educational definition: 'When sight is not good enough for learning by sighted methods' is one overall way of describing the condition. In babies one can use something more specific, e.g. 'without visually directed reaching', that is, when the baby does not look first and then reach out.

By the time school age is reached it is necessary to subdivide again into the blind and the partially sighted. This is less easy than it may seem, for no two children use their vision in the same way. Child A with a high level of intelligence and strong motivation will use his vision quite differently from child B who is less bright and more apathetic. In practice the decision usually rests on whether or not the child can learn to read using ink print. If this is not possible even with magnification, then the child is educated as one who is blind and learns Braille (see *Figure 7*).

CATEGORIES OF SIGHT

Having said all that, there remains a classification system which is in common use. It is based on the results of the familiar eye test in which one reads off a list of letters of gradually decreasing size, known as the Snellen types. The card is placed six metres away and if the smallest letters are seen comfortably one's vision is described as 6/6. If one has to go up a row, to letters twice as big, then vision is 6/12. In everyday terms this means that a normally sighted person can see the '6/12' row standing twelve metres away. Thus vision of 6/60 indicates that the child in question has to stand six metres from letters that a normally sighted child can see from 60 metres.

Partial sight

Most children in special schools for the partially sighted have vision of 6/18 or less. Again, one cannot draw hard and fast lines, I have known children with 6/12 in a special school and with 6/24 in ordinary education. At the other end of the scale 6/60 is the borderline between the partially sighted and the blind.

Blindness

6/60 is a borderline; generally 3/60 or less is a measure which indicates blindness. Some children have some vision but not enough to see a Snellen card. For them categories are as follows:

1. C.F. Counts fingers at varying distances from the eyes.

2. H.M. Hand movements can be perceived at a distance of 6 inches or more.

3. P.L. Perception of light.

4. Total blindness.

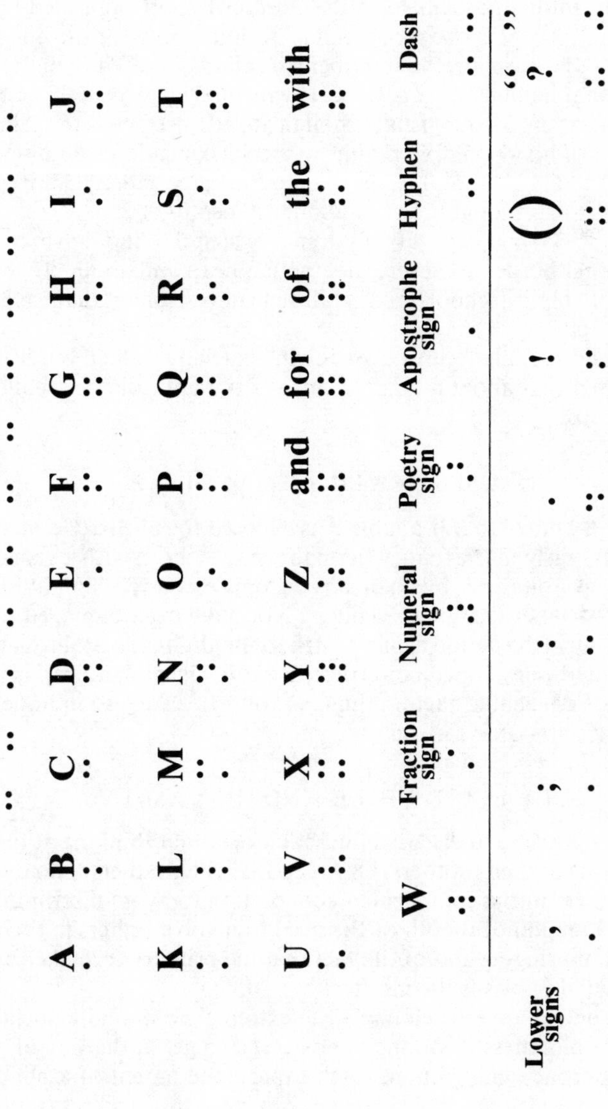

A B C D E F G H I J

K L M N O P Q R S T

U V W X Y Z and for of the with

Fraction sign Numeral sign Poetry sign Apostrophe sign Hyphen Dash

Lower signs , ; : . ! ( ) ?

Figure 7 The Braille alphabet

FREQUENCY

It is not possible to be certain about the numbers of visually handicapped children because registration is not universal. The pattern, though, as shown in the Vernon Report published by the DES in 1972 is one of a steadily declining rate for the blind and an increase in the number of blind children with an additional handicap. This Report, which concerned itself with the education of the visually handicapped, predicted that the number of blind children requiring special education would settle to a total of about 0.9 per 10,000. Partially sighted children would, it was thought, fall to about 2.0 per 10,000.

About 35 per cent of children registered blind have the additional burden of severe mental handicap and about 50 per cent of blind school-aged children have some additional handicap.

No comparable figures exist for the partially sighted but it is estimated that about a quarter suffer from appreciable second handicaps.

CAUSES OF VISUAL HANDICAP

It is well known that if a mother is exposed to rubella (German measles) early in pregnancy her baby may be born with a visual handicap. But this is by no means the only cause. The condition might be inherited, or the child might have been damaged in some way in the period around birth, or might have sustained an accident. In developed countries far more visual handicap is a result of congenital factors than is proportionately so in undeveloped parts of the world.

THE BLIND CHILD AND HIS FAMILY

It is not possible to discuss blind babies without thinking at the same time of their mothers. Or, of course, their fathers; I do not want to get into a complicated convolution to avoid discrimination. I am mindful both of the need to involve fathers in their child's upbringing and of the fact that the primary caretaker of most blind babies is the mother.

The news is overwhelming – the extreme emotional associations of blindness mentioned above tend to get in the way of a cool approach and who on earth expects the parent of a blind baby to stay cool anyway? Having said that, and the matter of parental emotions is discussed in more detail in Chapter 2, the need for action from parents remains at the forefront of planning. In a way this can be consoling for a mother because she can do something, a great deal in fact, to help offset her child's condition. The first step is to put the family in touch with the local assessment team for the visually impaired. Unfortunately not all local authorities have this service and the next step is to put the family in touch with the Royal National Institute for the Blind (RNIB) who have a team of advisers travelling all over the country to help parents at home. Excellent though this service is, there is only a handful of advisers and they cannot make frequent visits. Other professionals may be at hand to supplement the work of the RNIB, and the Institute publishes a couple of first-rate booklets for parents. The following few sections owe much to these booklets and to the work of several psychologists, notably Norah Gibbs and Doris Wills. None of these sections is meant to be complete, for them to be so it would be necessary to take far more space than is available. Instead the aim is to present examples under each heading to give an idea of the type of work necessary.

BONDING AND THE BLIND BABY

The blind baby does not return a smile, does not respond to his mother's change in facial expression, does not, indeed, respond at all in the way many parents expect him to. The result is that many mothers find bonding quite difficult. (For a fuller discussion of the principle of bonding see Chapter 4.) As one psychologist put it, 'Falling in love with a baby isn't automatic, it's cemented.' With blind babies there needs to be a good deal of knowledge to enable the cement to set.

GENERAL PRINCIPLE OF WORK WITH THE BLIND CHILD

The general principle is that the parent has to be far more of a teacher to a blind than to a non-handicapped child. Left to themselves blind children are likely to remain relatively immobile, resisting change, and seeming to be backward. (The fact that so many of them are mentally handicapped is an additional burden to the parent at this stage. It does not, however, mean that help should not be offered to a blind child even if he is retarded as well.)

The reason for this general principle is twofold. In the first place they are without the major means of gaining information and so this has in part to be made up for. In the second, they do not see others walking, drawing, throwing balls, and running and so miss a large part of the stimulus to action that comes from imitation. These are extreme statements, referring fully only to the totally blind. The need to encourage children to use what sight they have left is immense.

The developmental sequences of blind children are the same as those found in the sighted but they are, in some areas, slower to emerge. For example, blind babies reach out to a sound at about nine months, compared to the normal child who does this at about four months.

SOME KEY POINTS FOR THOSE WORKING WITH BLIND BABIES AND YOUNG CHILDREN

Movement

Blind babies often go still when their mother approaches. This is not a sign of rejection; it is an indication that the baby is concentrating.

Sighted babies lift their head and later try to walk because they can see that this is of value. The blind baby needs encouragement.

Blind babies' hands are often 'dead'. The baby needs help to find them, perhaps with a bell on one wrist at a time.

Sound and language

Blind people do not develop superhuman hearing but they do learn to use their hearing more efficiently than most sighted people.

Background noise is bad: radios, televisions, and record players should be turned off unless they are being listened to.

Blind babies need conversation partly to help them learn to

talk and partly to enable them to keep track of where the other person is. It is helpful to keep up a running commentary, reinforced with frequent touching, to provide babies with a sense of security.

No blind child should be touched without a prior warning word or sound.

As a sighted child builds up a vocabulary of words, so a blind one must develop a vocabulary of sounds as well. These include footsteps, differences in the sound of water from a tap and from a teapot, and other everyday sounds we take for granted.

Cause and effect can be taught via sound, for example by having a toy which makes a noise when shaken.

The meanings of some words have to be taught carefully, especially those like ceiling which a child will not normally touch.

FEEDING

The blind baby does not take kindly to a change in diet. For him feeding is a more enclosed activity than for a sighted child, with none of the distractions of pictures on plates and cups or the sight of others eating at the same time. The result seems to be a more intense experience and a reluctance to try anything new. If this pattern sets in it is then difficult to get him to take different textures and he refuses to chew. At this time mothers often feel reluctant to insist on change, because they do not want to make their children unhappy. The longer it is put off the harder it will be to get the child into a varied diet and an early gradual, start is recommended.

An early start to finger feeding is also recommended, say at about six to seven months. At first it will be messy, at first he will have to be taught to feel around for something he has dropped, and at first he may reject anything but rather strong tastes and smells. But it is a step towards independence.

VISUAL TRAINING

For the 90 per cent of registered blind children who have some residual sight there is a lot of point in working with the vision that remains. This will not restore sight but it will enable the child to make full use of what he has. This should, however, be undertaken only after the broad outlines of the approach have been discussed with whoever has medical responsibility for the child. As with all the sections in this part of the book, my aim is to give an indication of the work that can be done. Further details can be found in the RNIB pamphlets, from which the following suggestions have been taken.

Visual attention: string a wide elastic strip across the cot and hang on to it brightly coloured objects, e.g. a rattle or shatter proof Christmas decorations.

Fixation: fix a shiny windmill close by him in a place where it will spin easily.

Tracking: move a coloured torch from one side to another and then up and down.

MANNERISMS

Nine months is a crucial period for the blind baby, it is then that reacting to sound often begins as does another characteristic, much less welcome, known as 'blindisms'. These mannerisms are most distressing: eye poking, rocking while sitting, twirling around when standing up, flapping hands. The children look mad to those with no understanding and autistic to those with a little knowledge. The explanation is not that the child is mad, or bad, rather he is providing himself with a pleasurable stimulation. All children need movement and the blind child's movement is often restricted.

Observation has shown that blindisms occur most frequently when the child seems to have nothing else to do. Telling him to stop has no effect in the long term, it is better to provide an alternative activity. Better still is to try to prevent the mannerisms developing or getting a firm hold in the first place.

TOYS

Play has not been given a separate category because much of what has been discussed already could be included under this heading and in any case the subject is discussed in a general way elsewhere in this book (Chapter 6).

But toys for the blind child are something of a special case. His first toys are similar to those of a sighted child although they may be simpler, brighter, with more sound-making attachments. Later, just like a sighted child, he will enjoy playing with everyday objects rather than toys, a wooden spoon and a saucepan for example. But he will play in a slightly different way, seeking more often to produce a noise. Paper will be scrunched up for the feel and the sound, boxes will be rattled.

Models are taken to much later by the blind than the sighted. A model car, for example means nothing to a child who has never seen a full-size one, and a model cat has nothing of the feel, smell, or sound of a real animal. This does not mean, though, that children should not be encouraged to play pretend games, they can still have a tea party but with a real, small tea set rather than a dolls' one.

As the child gets older so he will develop interests of his own and universal rules cannot be applied. A Toy Library is invaluable at this stage, not only to avoid having to buy expensive toys which may not be used but also to swap ideas with other parents.

And as he gets older so he will learn to put his toys away, always in the same place so that they can be found again. Later this will generalize to other possessions.

THE PARTIALLY SIGHTED CHILD

To some small extent the points discussed above apply also to the partially sighted child, the child who has a visual handicap but who can learn using ink print rather than Braille. But not fully and not for all partially sighted children, for there is far greater variation in sight among them than there is among the registered blind. I have known partially sighted girls who could produce exquisite needlework and boys who played as good a game of football as most sighted peers. (They were not so good at cricket, though.) This variation means that generalizations about the partially sighted are as difficult to make as about any other group of handicapped children.

The emotions aroused are different from those elicited by the blind. The child peering about, head held forward with rather hesitant movement is not a figure of pity; he is often a figure of fun. Even if he wears thick glasses it is usually assumed that he can see and so when he bumps into someone else this is

often construed as carelessness or stupidity. They pass as
sighted; they fail like the blind.

The degree to which partial sight is a disability is often
questioned. To read some of the literature one might think that
it is not really much of a problem, for the difficulties described
in work with the blind do not exist. To read other examples in the
literature the problems are immense, especially those concerned
with education where highly complex technical aids are seen as
necessary. To read yet a third sort of book is even more daunting
because it becomes clear that very little research has been carried
out in this area.

Really, though, to ask whether partial sight is a true disability
– as blindness undoubtedly is – is to be rather naive. And I say
that having in the past posed it myself. It is naive because of the
enormous variation in visual handicap and because of the high
incidence of secondary handicaps found among the partially
sighted. There is a continuum from the otherwise healthy child
with myopia and a visual acuity of 6/18 to a child with cerebral
palsy and optic atrophy and a visual acuity of 6/60. Both might
be classified as partially sighted yet their problems are poles
apart.

There is, however, one generalization which can be made, and
that is to do with eye strain. Up to about 1960 children were not
allowed to use their eyes for close work for more than thirty
minutes, after which they had to have a rest period. This is now
seen to be unnecessary; residual vision should be used to the full.

EDUCATION

Until recently educational provision for the visually handicapped was a relatively simple matter: the blind went to boarding schools, sometimes well before they were five; the partially
sighted had a wider range of provision with more day schools
available; and both groups had an opportunity to go for a
grammar education at secondary stage.

Now the position is less clear cut. In the first place there has
been a strong movement away from boarding schools, not only
for the blind three-year-old but for all children. This has led to
an increase in flexibility: one may now find more young blind
children in day schools for the partially sighted, and the
Warnock Report's emphasis on needs rather than categories is

likely to see this pattern extended. A few, a very few, blind children attend ordinary schools, with their special school acting as a resource centre. But the selective schools remain and the general pattern of blind boarding, with the partially sighted having more choice, remains. Much depends on where one lives. There is always more choice in a densely populated area simply because there are more children to provide demands on an education service.

THE OUTLOOK

Some blind and partially sighted children go on to higher education, others may transfer to one of the vocational assessment centres which offer a link between the rather protected world of school and the open world. Only about 40 per cent of blind adults available and capable of work were, in 1979, employed and there has been some criticism of vocational training and indeed of special school standards. The fact remains, though, that Britain has the highest proportion of blind people in open employment of any country in the world.

Marriage is far from impossible. The RNIB publishes a pamphlet of advice for the blind mother. Blind men, however, more commonly marry sighted partners than do blind women. The blind do marry each other as well, although this is less common than marriage between the blind and the sighted. The strain on the children of a blind couple can be great, for they carry responsibility far beyond the normal. Evidence from Sweden suggests, though, that much depends on the maturity of the parents and whether or not they have additional handicaps.

Two closing comments, both from blind men. The first, Harvey Morris, has written, 'As a blind man, the simple fact that I cannot drive a car puts me immediately at a tremendous disadvantage. In lodgings a landlady will often make no special provision for a blind man, such as leaving the furniture always in the same place. If there is a lot of noise where he is working, he is more or less completely isolated.' The second is from Ted Bailey, a neighbour of mine who has been blind from birth. He said, 'I've had a good life – but it's been hard work.'

Part Three

18   The child with a life-threatening condition

'How much is a mother expected to bear?'

This question was asked by a mother who lost two children. Quoted in *The Care of the Child Facing Death* (1974), edited by Lindy Burton, it sums up the feelings of many people that losing a child is near to the unbearable. I say 'near to' because most families find that with help they can eventually bear the idea. The child is never forgotten, the pain is never forgotten, life is not the same as it would have been, but it can become bearable.

Until the end of the nineteenth century a child's death was a commonplace event in all social classes. Today, although the total annual number may seem high (there were 11,917 deaths under the age of fifteen in England and Wales in 1976) it is proportionately tiny, about 0.1 per cent and the overwhelming expectation is that children will live. We are, therefore, badly equipped to deal with death when it does occur. Medical and nursing staff, particularly those in junior positions, are especially vulnerable because their training is coupled with society's anticipation, leading them to see themselves as people who cure, not people who help others to end their lives. This problem is discussed fully in the introduction to a collection of interviews with bereaved people compiled by Rosamund Richardson (*Losses: Talking about Bereavement*). Several of those who talk about their experiences have lost children and their memories highlight many of the difficulties that are discussed in the rest of this chapter.

FAMILIES

Everything that has been written about families in Chapter 2 applies to those whose child may die, only more so. As the paediatrician Simon Yudkin has written, 'At no time does the personality of the family unit reflect itself so clearly' (Yudkin, 1967). The rest of this section has, therefore, been written on the assumption that Chapter 2 has been read. What follows is more in the nature of a commentary on problems from the standpoint of a family facing a death.

When parents first hear a diagnosis of handicap or chronic illness they often seem to go through stages of mourning, as though they had a sense of loss of a well child. The diagnosis of a life-threatening condition frequently brings the same reaction, for families mourn an actual death in anticipation. As the social worker Margaret Atkin has noted (Atkin, 1974), this is worst of all for those couples who see themselves as parents first and spouses second, especially when an only child is involved, for they face not only the loss of a child but also the loss of their own identity. The result of anticipatory mourning is a conflict: on the one hand parents feel they are withdrawing from the child who is, in prospect, dead already; on the other hand they desperately want to care for him. Conflict of this sort can be expressed in anger, parents guiltily finding themselves wishing the child was already dead or had never been born. It is no wonder that death is often seen as a relief when it does finally come.

Equally heightened by the possibility of death is the inability to anticipate the future. Medical advances in the last twenty years or so have brought not only increased hope but increased uncertainty. Will he live to be ten, or twenty, or twenty-five? Perhaps he will live long enough for a cure to be found? Perhaps he will die next month. The father of a child with acute lympho-blastic leukaemia, given a 50 per cent chance of surviving for at least five years, said to me that he felt he would be psycho-logically more settled if he knew that she was going to die within twelve months. Then, he said, he would be able to sort out his feelings. I am not sure that all parents would agree with him, but he made a fair point.

A sense of isolation is frequently felt by parents of any sick or handicapped child; the feeling is acute among those whose child's life is threatened. Some parents bring isolation on themselves, they refuse ever to tell anyone else the name of their child's illness, preferring either to lie or to be evasive and say 'he's got a weak chest' or 'he's a bit anaemic'. I have even met parents who invented a name not known to medical science. One of the reasons the parents do this is to avoid the look of horror and embarrassment that greets words like tumour, cancer, and leukaemia. But in avoiding that response they also avoid a frank discussion of their child, and their isolation is increased.

But one must not try to push parents to the other extreme. Very few can totally accept the inevitability of their child's death and the refusal to name the disease may be part of a defence against the whole truth. Such defences are not only common they may be necessary to maintain a parent's sanity, for without a tiny spark of hope a person can be destroyed. No one, no matter how good his intentions, has any right to take away that spark.

Brothers and sisters have their own problems. If the sick child is younger the well children may feel guilty at their earlier expressions of jealousy. If he is older they may re-live the resentment they felt at his having more privileges than they. If, tragically, they have the same condition they will watch the course of decline first in a brother or sister and then in themselves.

No matter how parents try not to favour one child they rarely succeed. One twelve-year-old said reflectively after his brother's death, 'Now I understand why dad took so many photos of Jimmy.' This boy had not been told how seriously ill his brother was, but at least he had been told of his death. I once had to see an eight-year-old whose brother had died three years before. He still thought that his brother was in hospital, or to be more accurate, his parents continued to tell him that his brother was still in hospital.

CHILDREN THEMSELVES

There is a perennial problem of what to tell children. In part this is a question of how much to tell them about their condition, for example how much should one tell a boy with muscular dystrophy about sexual dysfunction? In part it is simply whether one should tell the child the name of his illness. In some American hospitals the medical staff insist on all children knowing the name, in most British centres the decision is left to the parents. Some illnesses are easier to explain than others. The cause and treatment of renal failure are so closely related that explanations are both essential and easy to give. Leukaemia is a different matter, for children cannot always see the connection between their treatment and any feeling of being ill. In fact they often enter hospital feeling relatively well and leave feeling ill.

Sooner or later children seem to pick up something of their parents' emotions and something of the nature of their condition. They may discover something by accident, like the boy who read a letter addressed to his mother in which a reference was made both to him and his illness. They may pick up an ill-digested half knowledge, which will give rise to more worry than would a full understanding. But, for it is arrogant of commentators to be certain on such matters, they may sail through life, safe in their ignorance.

The child's inability to understand the gravity of his illness is a reason often given by parents for saying very little to him. Another reason is that children do not appear to be particularly interested – at least they rarely ask questions which embarrass their parents. It is true that children hardly ever ask outright, 'Am I going to die?' But this does not mean that their thoughts are not running on this topic. A crucial point in such deliberations is whether or not the child has a fully developed concept of what dying means.

A child's concept of death does not develop overnight, rather it forms over a period of time from a first, vague awareness in which it is confused with sleep, through an association with coffins and burials to a full understanding of the irreversibility of the final state. Research in this area is scant. Work with healthy children, for example that of Sylvia Anthony in *The Discovery of Death in Childhood and After* (1971), suggests that a partial realization rarely occurs before the age of five, with the turning point in the move towards a fully formed concept coming at seven or eight. Only at the age of nine or ten does the concept of death as adults know it really take root.

Such suggestions can be questioned. Anthony's work was carried out in the 1930s, in a time of peace, and it would be unwise to generalize from work with healthy children to conclusions about the fatally sick. A recent book on the sick child's knowledge of death is *The Private Worlds of Dying Children* (1978) by Myra Bluebond-Langner. The author reports on a study of 40 children aged three to nine years seen in an American hospital. 18 children were followed intensively and the most significant finding was that both adults and children joined in a 'mutual pretence' that death was not imminent. This defence was seen to be a shield against psychological pain. If this study is shown to be true in other settings the implications for the management of dying children are enormous, for it would appear that children are carrying a much heavier load than has, in some quarters, been imagined.

BEHAVIOURAL RESULTS

Children who acquire a life-threatening illness have a set of prior experiences different from those who suffer from a congenital condition, as was discussed in Chapter 3. In their early years they were proud of gaining mastery over their body and then, with increasingly serious an illness, their bodily control diminishes and frustration and anger set in. They become, as Bluebond-Langner pointed out, like very old people, with nothing to look forward to. And they are surrounded by an emotionally upset family.

There is no one characteristic behaviour pattern but there are several broad types. One is withdrawal, which may be accompanied by regression. The child clings to his parents, stops wanting to see his friends and demands to be babied. Another is aggression: the child fights with anyone in sight and may attack even himself by refusing to accept treatment, ripping out a drip or spitting out tablets. This seems often to be a disguised attack on his parents for allowing him to get so ill. Bianca Gordon, a psychotherapist writing in Lindy Burton's book, tells of an eleven-year-old girl whose last words to her mother were 'I hate you'. Other children try excessively to compete, to show that they can still manage despite what the doctors say. And some children are unnaturally good. Whatever the behaviour the key factor to look for is sudden change, for that in itself is a danger signal.

WAYS OF HELPING

Before the child dies

Cecily Saunders, who has cared for many terminally ill people, has written that the dying child needs to have 'a climate of security'. Indeed, the whole family needs such a climate for this is a time when they feel most cut off from everything they have come to see as predictable and normal. The key to help is security, predictability, and normality.

Help can be given in a number of ways. One is to ensure that families are, as far as possible, prepared for what will happen. Many parents are afraid, for example, to ask exactly how a child will die. Linked with this provision is the general principle of ensuring that each family has at least one person, perhaps more than one, who knows them as individuals. Time and time again I have heard parents say how much they appreciate the fact that Dr X always recognizes them in the hospital corridor and always addresses their child by name.

Parents need an opportunity to talk to someone about their feelings without thinking that the person they are talking to will be upset, embarrassed, or bored. A doctor may meet this need but parents are reluctant to take up scarce medical time. Sometimes they can talk to each other, or to a friend, neighbour, or relation; but not always. A social worker can often fill the role required without arousing a feeling on the part of the parents that they are imposing on another's time. Other parents benefit more from sharing their experiences with those in a similar position and for them a parents' group, preferably led by a professional, is of great value. What seems important in this context is that a wide variety of opportunities be given, for not only will different families have different needs, each family itself changes as the child's illness progresses.

Perhaps of equal importance, but more rarely offered, is counselling for other members of the family and for the children themselves. This seems often to be reserved for those who show overt behaviour disturbances: you have to be naughty to get help.

Even more rarely discussed is the need to provide support for the medical and nursing staff or for teachers. The care of a dying child is stressful whoever one is, and the best support to parents can only be given when staff themselves can function as efficiently as possible.

Many parents feel that normality is regained once they can do something for their child even if it is no more than washing, dressing and feeding him. For some, of course, the burden is much heavier and may involve several hours physiotherapy a day. The normality comes because the parent is behaving like a parent in providing care. But this can be gained at a price, for if the child's health deteriorates the parent who has taken so much care may blame herself for failing to do even more.

An extension of behaving like a parent is the provision of discipline. The over-indulged child, given everything he wants and a lot more that he does not want, does not feel normal, i.e. like his friends, and will rebel. Much of the behaviour disturbance mentioned already in this chapter seems to be a cry from the child for control. The parent who can impose limits is able to provide just the security that the child needs. (This is, as parents have so often told me, easier said than done.)

One relatively easy way to provide a normal environment for a child is to send him to school, preferably an ordinary rather than a special school. The view sometimes held, that if a child is going to die by the time he is twelve there is no point in educating him, does not seem to me to stand up. Children expect to go to school, no matter how much they may complain. What is more, if they are going to die at twelve then school life will have been virtually their whole life, so it is doubly important to ensure that it is of the highest possible quality.

When the child dies

Death can never be predicted with certainty. But there are times when a prediction can be made with near enough certainty and decisions have to be made about the child's last days. If possible it is usually better if he can be at home. This is partly because his parents can be with him and with other members of the family all the time; if he remains in hospital it is hard to leave him even for ten minutes. It is partly becuase parents can then feel free to remain with the child's body during the hours just after his death, helping to lay him out. In hospital this is also possible, but parents may feel that they cannot just sit by a dead child's bedside there because they think they are getting in the way.

As some parents are afraid to ask how a child is likely to die, so they are afraid to ask, or even to think about, what they will be doing around this time. It may be necessary for professional staff to help them overcome such fears.

After the child's death

One of the best ways for a hospital or school staff to help a family at this time is to give them an opportunity to return to visit the staff. So often parents feel that all contact has ceased once their child is no longer a patient or pupil. Yet hospital becomes a central part in the life of many families and they feel an additional sense of abandonment if they can no longer visit. Some parents return on a child's birthday, or the anniversary of his death. Others give something as a token of their child; one mother donated an old armchair to a hospital playcentre because her daughter had been unable to stand during the last months of her illness and the playcentre chairs had become very important to her.

If parents have become accustomed to being visited, say by a health visitor or district nurse, this contact should be ended gradually rather than suddenly at the child's death. An occasional call, even after several months, is usually greatly appreciated.

A consistent thread that runs through all discussions on parental needs is the value of being able to meet someone else who has had a similar experience. In this context the Society of Compassionate Friends, founded in 1969, offers immediate help (see address list).

Because we are so little accustomed to mourning a child we do not know what to expect of a bereaved family. Families must mourn, yet they sometimes worry because they think that their feelings are somehow abnormal. Knowing what is commonly experienced can be a help at times of severe distress, a point considered at some length by Simon Stephens in the concluding chapter of Lindy Burton's *The Care of the Child Facing Death*. Common reactions include:

Shock and numbness.

Sleeplessness, loss of appetite, general apathy.

Guilt: 'If only I had . . . '

Preoccupation with the dead child's image, he is 'seen' in a crowd or 'heard' on the stairs.

It may seem strange that a whole chapter has been written about death with virtually no mention of religion. This omission is not because I underestimate its value for some people: I know one mother who has been sustained for years by her belief in Christianity. But I also know others for whom their professed faith has been of little apparent value and I follow the thoughts of Simon Yudkin, the paediatrician I have already quoted. He pointed out that religion is a personal and family matter; it is not justifiable for professional staff to impose their own beliefs on child or parent.

19   Asthma

DEFINITION

This condition has been known for at least 5,000 years, the word 'asthma' coming from the Greek meaning 'panting' or 'gasping'. And pant and gasp is just what asthmatics do. They sit, hunched up, often with stiffened arms, neck and shoulders, gasping for breath, fighting what seems to be an internal battle with their lungs.

The essential difficulty they have is not simply with breathing in general, it is specifically with breathing out. What happens in asthma is this: the air passages in the lung (the bronchial tubes) become narrow during the attack. The result is that air cannot be driven out of the lungs properly in time to take another breath in and the lungs become blown up.

TYPES OF ASTHMA

Asthma used to be divided into types, depending on what it was associated with. It is now generally accepted that nearly all asthma is associated with an allergy of one sort or another (see below under 'Causes') and earlier attempts at subdividing, e.g. according to an association with eczema or with hay fever, were misleading.

Another, more acceptable, way of dividing asthma into types is by severity. It may be mild, coming infrequently and lasting for only an hour or so, or it may be very severe, with attacks going on, in the most extreme form, for several days. Death from asthma in childhood is rare but not unknown.

FREQUENCY

Asthma is the most common handicapping disease among children in Great Britain and it has been estimated that up to one child in twenty suffers from it to some extent.

CAUSES

Despite its long history and the number of sufferers the causes of asthma are not fully understood. It is known that some children are allergic to certain substances. These substances include pollen, house dust and certain kinds of food. If a child who is allergic to one or more of these is exposed to whatever it is he is allergic to, his body reacts more violently than that of a normal child and certain chemicals are released within the body, leading to physical symptoms. In some children these symptoms are found in the nose (hay fever) some have them in the eyes (allergic conjunctivitis) and others have them in the lungs (asthma).

But an attack can also be brought on by undue exercise, by too much laughing, which is a form of exercise, and by stress. It was observations of this past point, that asthma can be brought on by stress, that led many people to make the mistake of thinking that psychological factors cause the condition.

PSYCHOLOGICAL FACTORS

Some doctors, but not all, describe asthma as a psychosomatic condition. A loose explanation of this phrase is that it means that 'it's all in the mind', i.e. the physical symptoms are directly caused by psychological reasons. Until recently it was fashionable to put forward the following neat explanation of the cause of asthma in childhood: it arose from a child's fear of being separated from his mother. This mother was seen as being outwardly over-protective but inwardly rejecting. This, and similar theories, have now been examined scientifically and have been found wanting. There is no evidence at all that psychological factors *on their own* cause asthma.

But even if we discount some of the wilder theories about rejecting mothers we should not totally ignore the part that emotions do play, not in the cause but in the course of the illness. It is now agreed that excitement, perhaps over a Christmas party, or stress, perhaps over an exam at school, can bring on an attack. The point is, though, that the child must have a physical tendency towards asthma in the first place. It follows from this that an important part of the management of asthmatic children is the reduction of undue stress. This will be dealt with more fully under 'Management' below.

More than Sympathy

MANAGEMENT

Long-term care

The most important physical way of preventing asthma is to try to eliminate anything to which the child is allergic. This may lead to the removal of feather pillows, wool blankets, and even some pets. Some children benefit from injections of a tiny amount of what they are allergic to, in order that they may build up an immunity.

Psychological ways of preventing an attack centre round the need to reduce the amount of stress experienced by the child. One cannot expect him to live totally in a world without excitement or stress, although some parents do go to considerable lengths to keep a child calm. I know of one boy whose parents always pretended, on December 24th, that Christmas Day was two days away in order that he should not get worked up. But one can observe a child to see if there is some pattern about his behaviour. Perhaps he starts to cough and then to wheeze when his parents are quarrelling, perhaps he seems worse when there are certain lessons in school. Quite often skilled professional help is needed to unravel this kind of pattern and then to do something about it. But half the battle is being aware of the forces that might be operating.

Management of an attack

Once an attack has started it is essential to relax the muscles of the bronchial tubes as quickly as possible. A mild attack may respond to nothing more sophisticated than the child sitting quietly sipping some warm water. More serious episodes usually respond to drugs, either in tablet form or from an inhaler. Inhalers work very quickly and can be dangerous if used too often or too much. **Medical advice must be sought by anyone who is responsible for a child using an inhaler.**

The psychological part of treatment is no simple matter. Some parents react strongly to an attack and their children soon learn that there is much to be gained by having, or prolonging, wheezing and coughing. Suddenly everyone drops whatever else they were doing and pays attention to the child, who is transformed into a patient. It need not even be a very subtle gain: I heard recently of one group of children who persuaded their teacher that their asthma meant that they had to spend every afternoon resting and watching television. Unfortunately the advice of 'don't be too nice to him' is easy to understand, but much harder to put into practice.

Other parents, though, reject their child, in which case advice about not being too nice is misplaced. One constant fact seems to be that it helps if one can enable children to express anxieties openly, rather than using asthma as a vehicle. This requires skilled intervention; the adult who says, 'Tell me what is worrying you' is likely to be met with nothing but silence. Often this silence is taken to mean that nothing is worrying the child and an opportunity to provide lasting help has been missed.

THE 'ASTHMATIC PERSONALITY'

Just as it used to be thought that there was a person called 'the asthma-producing mother' so it was believed that people who have asthma share certain characteristics. This view was put forward by a number of people, but their argument was weakened by the fact that they did not agree among themselves as to the nature of the characteristics that asthmatics were supposed to have. As happens so often to theories of this kind, when a large, representative group was studied it became clear that asthmatics vary as much as everyone else.

Two points, though, remain. Mothers of asthmatic children are more anxious than mothers of the non-asthmatic, and asthmatic children are, in some cases, more disturbed than their non-handicapped counterparts. Neither of these points is surprising, since both mother and child are subjected to quite frightening experiences. It is interesting to note in this context that the worse the asthma the greater the disturbance is likely to be. This is not so with most other handicaps or illnesses. The picture is also put into perspective when it is realized that neither the mothers' anxiety nor the children's disturbance is any greater than that found in other groups of handicapped or sick children.

INTELLIGENCE AND ATTAINMENT

There is a commonly held belief that asthmatic children are both more intelligent and do better in school than others. Before the late 1960s this was a view held in faith rather than being based on fact, and even now there is some uncertainty. Putting together what is known, it seems reasonable to say that asthmatic children do appear to be more intelligent than the average child, but their school work is, if anything, below average. The research that has been done in these areas is, however, thin, and one cannot be certain on either conclusion.

THE OUTLOOK FOR THE ASTHMATIC CHILD

Some children grow out of their asthma, some do not. Some sporting activities, cross-country running or rugby for example, are not usually possible. But a boy can play football in goal and both sexes should be encouraged to swim.

Some occupations are obviously not suitable, it would be silly to expect someone allergic to pollen to work as a gardener. But a wide range of jobs is available and the future is far from bleak.

20   Cystic fibrosis

From a father: 'I think we are living in hell now; anything after this will be heaven.'

From a child: 'Do they have physiotherapy in heaven?'

DEFINITION

To most people 'cystic fibrosis' conveys the fact that someone has a relatively rare illness, and that is about all. Sometimes it is confused with fibrositis, although in fact the two are quite different. Cystic fibrosis is a life-threatening condition that affects both the lungs and the digestive system.

First, the lungs: we all have a substance in our lungs called mucus. It coats the bronchial tubes and helps in the expulsion of germs and dust. In a healthy person it is thin and slippery but in cystic fibrosis it is thick and sticky, tending to block up certain parts of the body, for example the smaller bronchial tubes. The result is a persistent cough, difficulty in breathing, and a greater than average vulnerability to chest infection. Before the disease was identified in 1939 such children were usually described as 'chesty' and often died from pneumonia in infancy.

Second, the digestive system: one of the parts of the body to be blocked in cystic fibrosis is the pancreatic gland, which is involved in the production of digestive juices. Without these juices the body cannot properly absorb fats and starch. The result is that they are both excreted in foul smelling stools. Rather more serious than the smell is the consequence that without absorbing fat and starch the child fails to thrive.

One of the distinctive symptoms of cystic fibrosis is the high salt content in sweat, the child tastes salty, especially in hot weather.

There is a tendency towards an all round slower physical growth, puberty comes later than in most children, and boys are usually smaller than average. Girls can sometimes have children although boys are generally infertile, while maintaining normal sexual functioning.

But not all children are affected to the same extent. Some can manage more exercise than others; some need more intensive treatment than others; some need to be on a diet, others do not.

FREQUENCY

Estimates on how many children suffer from the disease vary, the most commonly quoted figure being one in 2,000. One American study has suggested that as many as one third of all children with cystic fibrosis are not diagnosed, so present estimates must be regarded with caution.

CAUSES

The exact nature of the physical fault is unknown. It is an inherited condition and is passed on to a child from both parents. If the gene is received from one parent only then the child will not have the illness but will be a 'carrier', that is will be able to pass it on to his or her child. It has been estimated that about one in twenty-five people in North West Europe are carriers. (The condition is less common elsewhere.) When both parents are carriers it is not certain that the child will inherit cystic fibrosis, but the chances are high: about one in four.

TREATMENT

There is no cure. Among those diagnosed in childhood most do not live to be adult, although some are now still alive in their twenties. This does not mean that there is no treatment, indeed for some children there is a very vigorous regime which, if successfully carried out, can do much to improve the quality of the child's life.

The lungs

There are two aspects here, the first being keeping them relatively clear in order that the child may breathe freely. This involves close co-operation between child, parent and physiotherapist and may take up to three half-hour sessions of physiotherapy a day. Parents are taught how to treat their child so that the sticky mucus moves from smaller to larger tubes and children learn the best way to cough. Exercise is a great benefit, the more the better. Not all children can keep up with all games but this need not be a complete bar; it is better to play half a game of football than none at all.

The second aspect is the need to combat infections that may lead to permanent lung damage. Today antibiotics are a powerful weapon in this fight.

Smoking is dangerous.

Digestion

The pancreatic gland is not working and so all children have to take a replacement substance before every meal. It can be in powder, capsule or tablet form.

Some children also have to keep to a diet which is similar to that for people who are overweight: acceptable are lean meat and bacon, fish and eggs which may be given in larger than normal portions. Not acceptable are cake or pastry in any quantity, or fried foods unless they are prepared in a special oil.

PSYCHOLOGICAL FACTORS

Just before and just after the diagnosis

Unless the condition is diagnosed very early in the child's life, which happens in only a minority of cases, the parents are likely to undergo a particularly confidence-sapping period. They have a baby who looks normal, eats ravenously and yet does not thrive. Many parents seek advice and are told not to be fussy. In desperation they blame themselves, changing their feeding patterns wildly. This may go on for several months and by the time the diagnosis is made they lack confidence in their own ability to bring up a child.

When they learn that the cause is genetic, that is, it is 'their fault' that the child has cystic fibrosis, there is every chance that they will feel guilty as well as incompetent. When they come to realize that the condition is life-threatening they encounter all the problems that accompany such an outlook. (See Chapters 2 and 18 for a fuller discussion of all these points.)

THE PSYCHOLOGY OF MANAGEMENT

To outsiders the problems may seem slight. There the child is, running about just like anyone else, going to school just like anyone else. He coughs a bit and is rather fussy about his food, but these are not things to worry about are they?

In fact, as Lindy Burton has described in her book *The Family Life of Sick Children* (1975), the problems for child and parent are gigantic.

The knowledge that they, the parents, will have to do a lot of physiotherapy with children brings a sense of relief to many parents; at least and at last there is something positive which they can do. But soon the burden of the responsibility of this task takes over, for if the child becomes worse the parents are likely to blame themselves. Constant reassurance from physiotherapists is needed not only in a time of crisis but at all times, along with constant checking that parents have fully understood what they are supposed to be doing. The sense of responsibility for treatment also means that parents dare not be ill, or away from their child, for it is not easy to find someone else both able and prepared to take their place for up to three hours a day.

The spending of so much time on physical needs can lead to a neglect of a child's emotional needs. Like all sick and handicapped children, they can easily become dependent on their parents, staying rather young for their age. In the case of a child with cystic fibrosis the pull towards both dependence and childishness is all the greater partly because they are literally dependent on their parents for care, and partly because of the slower physical development that is characteristic of their growth. They too, can learn to use their treatment as a weapon, refusing sometimes to take tablets or to co-operate in physiotherapy. (See Chapters 2, 5, and 19 for a further discussion of these points.)

PRETENDING

Sometimes there is a pretence that the child does not have a serious illness, a pretence which is joined in by parents and child. The cough is explained by referring to asthma, or a permanent frog in the throat. Sometimes the pretence reaches the level that treatment is stopped, as though it is hoped that the illness will just go away in some magical way. Many of us have magical thoughts about all sorts of things, usually trivial; in the case of cystic fibrosis the results can be disastrous.

WAYS OF HELPING

Some of the difficulties faced by children and parents cannot fully be overcome. The prospect of death is not something that can be talked into insignificance. But much can be done by bringing everyone, parents, children and medical staff, into a partnership. What has been called by the American social worker J. Turk, 'the web of silence' can be broken. This means that one ensures that everyone understands what the treatment is all about. In conditions like cystic fibrosis this is both easier and more important than in many others because the illness and the treatment are both bound together and the child himself has to co-operate. Lindy Burton gives an example of bad communication when she tells of a mother who told her daughter that she was having physiotherapy because she had a mouse in her chest which had to be got out. Ways of sharing both information and worries are discussed in Chapter 10.

It helps also to develop a formula to explain the problems to neighbours or a child's school friends. Talk of genetics and pancreatic glands may be too much; an explanation using words like 'something wrong with the body's chemistry' is usually easier both to say and to understand.

EDUCATION

Children with cystic fibrosis are in the normal range of intelligence. This does not mean that none is subnormal any more than it means that none is very bright, it does mean, though, that they should receive as ordinary an education as possible. For many of them school is the only entirely ordinary place they go to, and contact with non-handicapped children is a great reassurance. Teachers must be informed of the nature of the condition, for few of them will have encountered it before.

Most school difficulties revolve around an understanding of a child's cough, the need to provide the right amount of exercise and to be careful over diet. None of these is beyond a good school. But if physiotherapy is needed during the day then attendance at a special school will probably be necessary. Home tuition is recommended only as a last resort.

THE OUTLOOK

Physically the outlook is double-edged. On the one hand the condition is life-threatening, on the other hand modern medical knowledge means that an increasing number of sufferers are able to live on into their twenties.

The range of work opportunities is determined more by the person's intelligence and personality, and the state of the market, than by their illness, although some jobs are unsuitable – for example those involving heavy manual labour. Studies by the American Cystic Fibrosis Foundation show that people are working as the following: engineer, filing clerk, advertising account executive, airline stewardess, supermarket manager, teacher, nurse, lawyer, and printer. Of 300 young people surveyed by the Foundation 93 per cent said that they were satisfied with their jobs and 74 per cent reported that their health caused them no difficulties at work.

The outlook is less certain to be so optimistic about marriage. But providing both partners know exactly what it is there is no reason why someone with cystic fibrosis should not marry. In 1978 the British C.F. Trust knew of nineteen children born to mothers who have the illness, only two of whom had cystic fibrosis themselves.

21   Heart disease

DEFINITION

The phrase 'heart disease' is generally used to cover any abnormal condition of the heart and major blood muscles. Symptoms include shortness of breath, chest pains, fatigue, and a blue tinge to the skin and finger nails. Growth may be retarded.

Heart murmurs are often confused with heart disease. A murmur is the sound produced by the circulation of the blood through the valves and chambers of the heart and, if diagnosed as functional (sometimes called 'innocent') gives rise to no anxiety. If, however, the murmur is organic there is an indication that a defect is present.

CAUSES

Most heart disease in childhood is congenital. The heart develops early, at about the end of the third week of embryonic life and a severe structural defect will be present at the end of the eighth week. Although there is a very slight tendency for heart disease to run in families the cause of most congenital defects remains unknown. Rubella and possibly other diseases contracted during pregnancy increase the probability and there is an association with some chromosomal abnormalities, Down's Syndrome being among the most common.

Some children acquire a defect. Rheumatic fever, for example, can damage the heart muscle and lead to the formation of scar tissue on a valve in the heart, thus preventing the valve from opening and closing properly.

FREQUENCY

About one child in 100 is born with a heart defect but one third have no symptoms and require no treatment.

TREATMENT

Many conditions give rise to symptoms during the first year of life, but in others the child does not show any signs until he is coming up for school age. There are also a number of conditions which require treatment before the child goes to school, even in the absence of any symptoms, to prevent further changes taking place in later life. It is important to remember that some of the commonest conditions improve spontaneously even if they had caused symptoms early in life.

Because the conditions are due to a structural abnormality an operation is frequently required to correct those defects that do not improve on their own. Before this can be undertaken one needs to know precisely what the defects are. At the present time this usually involves a major investigation in which a tube is inserted into the vein and then into the heart to measure the colour of the blood in the various chambers and to take pressures. During the same procedure special X-ray pictures can be taken following the introduction of a radio-opaque dye through the tube. These investigations are known as cardiac catheterization and angiocardiography and they are usually carried out under sedation. Only in very rare instances is a general anaesthetic needed.

Of those conditions which require an operation more than three quarters can be corrected by surgery and many of the rest can be partially corrected. These are figures that lead to justifiable optimism. It must not be forgotten that heart disease is still a life-threatening condition, particularly during the first few months of life.

MANAGEMENT

Medical advice must always be available to anyone having responsibility for a child with heart disease, for it is not possible to generalize about dangers or restrictions. However, it is easy to overprotect any sick child and those with heart problems are no exception. In particular mothers of young children should be reassured that crying does not cause either pain or strain to the heart. Most children can attend ordinary schools and lead more or less normal lives, and although some competitive games may be forbidden swimming and cycling need not be ruled out.

EDUCATION

Heart disease does not cause mental retardation. Even if a child is cyanosed (that is, if the blood lacks oxygen causing the blue tinge referred to above) enough oxygen reaches the brain to prevent damage unless he is unfortunate enough to have had a stroke. But some children do fall behind in school, partly because they tire easily and partly because they lose school time while receiving treatment. Severely cyanosed children are known to have a shorter attention span than a healthy child. It is not true, then, that an operation will make a child more clever; it may help him to make the most of his abilities.

THE OUTLOOK

Some adults have to undertake work which involves little physical effort; some women are advised against becoming pregnant. Others can anticipate a normal life. The concluding sentence of the British Heart Foundation's booklet for parents consists of four words: 'The future is bright'.

22 Leukaemia

Leukaemia is usually described as 'cancer of the blood'. To understand what this means one must have some idea of what blood is and what job it does.

Blood consists of a fluid part, plasma, which carries chemical substances vital to the body, and a solid part, cells, which circulate bathed in the plasma. It is with the cells that we are primarily concerned when discussing leukaemia.

There are three types of cell:

1. *The red*: their task is the circulation of oxygen to all tissues of the body.

2. *The white*: their main function is the combatting of infection. There are two main types of white cell: lymphoid and myeloid.

3. *Platelets*: they are essential for the arrest of bleeding.

A deficiency in red cells leads to anaemia and children become pale and listless.

A deficiency of white cells may lead to a lowered resistance to certain types of infection.

A deficiency of platelets leads to spontaneous bleeding and to excessive bleeding after injury; children may vomit blood, have nose bleeds or show excessive bruising.

Most of the cells mentioned above are manufactured in the bone marrow which has been described as the 'factory' for cells. Leukaemia is the result of a failure of control in this factory. What happens is that some cells fail to mature properly and collect within the bone marrow and the blood. They increase and thus crowd out the mature, properly functioning cells, leading to the deficiencies noted above.

There are several types of leukaemia, classified according to the type of white blood cell which is mainly affected. The two main types are *myeloid* and *lymphoid*, which can be further sub-divided into acute and chronic. The acute form is rapid in onset and nearly always leads to death within a few months if it is untreated; the chronic form is slower both in onset and in its course.

Different types of leukaemia affect different age groups. Leukaemia diagnosed in childhood is most likely to be acute lymphoblastic. Of 100 children, about eighty-five will have acute lymphoblastic leukaemia (A.L.L.) and about fifteen will have acute myeloid (A.M.L.). Chronic myeloid and other forms are very rare.

The diagnosis of leukaemia is not a straightforward matter and may take several days.

FREQUENCY

There is slight variation throughout the world, with an average of one child in 25,000 being diagnosed. The peak age for the onset of A.L.L. is between two and five years.

CAUSES

No definite cause has been found for leukaemia in humans although certain types of virus cause leukaemia in some animals. There is no evidence that it can be inherited, nor that it is in any way catching, and there seems to be no increased risk to a child born into a family one member of which has the disease.

Rather more is known about factors which predispose towards the development of leukaemia, notably radiation. The dropping of the atomic bombs in Japan led to a higher than usual rate of the condition among survivors and hospital staff working with radioactive materials used to be vulnerable; preventative measures are now taken.

'There is no evidence whatsoever to suggest that anything that parents have done or failed to do, during their child's life, has any bearing on the development of this disease, and parents should never feel that it is anyone's "fault" that leukaemia has developed in their child.' From *A Guide to Treatment and*

174 *More than Sympathy*

Care published by the Leukaemia Research Fund, London.
(See address list.)

TREATMENT

All forms of leukaemia can be treated but not all can be cured.
Some authorities are cautious about using the word 'cure' at all,
for medical knowledge has only recently advanced sufficiently
to enable us to begin to think in such terms. At the moment the
outlook for children with A.M.L. is still very poor. Present
evidence suggests that 40 per cent of children with A.L.L. will
survive for at least five years and three quarters of those who
survive for four and five years without evidence of disease may
never subsequently relapse.

The treatment of leukaemia in childhood involves a series of
procedures which are painful and distressing in themselves,
leading usually to unpleasant after effects. One of the ironies of
treatment is that children often come to hospital feeling quite
well and go home, after their treatment, feeling sick. Against all
this, though, must be placed the end results.

The treatment varies according to the type of disease but in the
most common, A.L.L., it is as follows, with possibly some
overlapping between stages:

1. Getting a child into remission

'Remission' is a term used to describe a state when the child's
blood and bone marrow are restored to apparent normality. The
key word here is 'apparent', for present tests are relatively crude
and it is always possible that some leukaemic cells continue to
work in the body undetected. This stage usually takes three to
four weeks, during which drugs are used to attack the leukaemic
cells. The aim of this chemotherapy (i.e. drug treatment) is to do
as much harm as possible to the leukaemic cells and as little
damage as possible to the normal cells. This involves a careful
balance, the use of several drugs and constant monitoring of
what is going on.

2. Central nervous system treatment

There are certain sites in the body where leukaemic cells can
exist, protected from the effects of drugs given in the usual way.

These 'sanctuaries' include the brain and the spinal cord. Recent work suggests that the testes may also be involved in this way. It is very important that such sanctuaries be treated as soon as the child is in remission. This next stage of treatment consists of a combination of radiotherapy and drugs administered to the spinal cord by lumbar puncture. This stage also takes three to four weeks to complete.

3. Maintenance

This involves further drug therapy, with the aim of maintaining remission and eradicating as completely as possible any remaining leukaemic cells. This stage usually lasts between two and three years. If leukaemic cells do grow again the child is in 'relapse' and further measures have to be taken.

Some parents become upset when they discover that their child is on a different drug regime from another, although both have the same type of leukaemia and both were diagnosed at the same time. The reason for this is that different combinations of drugs are being tried all the time in order to determine which is the most effective. Without direct comparisons of drugs progress in treatment could not be made and so 'clinical trials' are used both in Britain and in other countries, all of which co-operate in reporting results. It must be emphasized that the basic treatment is the same for all children, the differences between trials are relatively small and as soon as it is clear that one treatment is better than another then the better method is used for all children.

SIDE EFECTS OF TREATMENT

Each drug has its own side effects; parents and children soon learn to anticipate them. Four in particular figure largely: vomiting, mouth ulcers, constipation and irritability. Constipation responds to a mild laxative but vomiting and the change of mood have to be coped with as the family sees fit. It is essential that parents know of possible side effects, understanding that apparent naughtiness can be a result of a drug.

The side effects noted above are usually temporary. More important is the fact that nearly all the drugs currently used in treatment have an effect on the normal working of the bone marrow which means that the symptoms of deficiencies in cells described in the first section of this chapter are still, to some extent, likely to be present. Of the three noted there: anaemia, a tendency to bleed, and reduced resistance to infection, the last is by far the most important and the most difficult to treat. The result is that even childhood illnesses like chicken pox and measles become serious to the point of being life-threatening.

Everyone who has any responsibility for a child, and this includes teachers, must be aware of the danger from serious infection. **If the child has been in contact with measles or chicken pox medical help should be sought immediately**. Similarly, it is important to notify one's doctor if a child becomes unwell with a fever or any unusual symptoms. At times like this it is better to speak to a doctor before bringing the child into contact with other children with leukaemia.

The most dramatic side effect of radiotherapy is loss of hair which passes after a few months. A minority of patients vomit and about fifty per cent develop symptoms of sleepiness and lack of concentration about five or six weeks after radiotherapy has stopped. This does not mean that the child has relapsed, and the phase passes within a couple of weeks.

There are three possible long-term side effects of treatment, but knowledge of these is, at the moment, slight and they cannot be regarded as more than possible.

The first is subfertility or infertility. Irradiation of the testes will have an obvious effect on boys but even apart from this there is the possibility that the very large doses of drugs that have to be used will have a similar effect.

The second is retardation of growth and the delay of puberty. Children with leukaemia do become pubertal but experience at the moment is not sufficient to be certain about the possibility of a slight growth retardation in adulthood. This does not seem to be a very serious problem and it is possible that children will catch up on lost ground once treatment has ceased.

The third is the possibility of slightly lowered intelligence. There is no doubt that children with leukaemia fall into the normal range of intelligence but there is some evidence to suggest that their IQ levels and attainments in school fall slightly below those of healthy children. The precise cause of this is uncertain and as with every other aspect of treatment mentioned in this chapter, research is being carried out in this area in order to monitor effects.

THE PSYCHOLOGICAL EFECTS ON CHILD AND FAMILY

Many of the points discussed in Chapter 2 and 18 apply to parents, brothers and sisters, and children. There is the shock of diagnosis, the danger of spoiling, the possibility of apparently rejecting brothers and sisters, and the constant, nagging anxiety.

But in one way leukaemia is different from most other diseases: the outcome is, for the 80 per cent of children with A.L.L., uncertain. Looking at it one way one can say that there is an even chance of the child living for at least five years and quite possibly for much longer. This is a hopeful picture compared to that of thirty years ago when one per cent of all children with leukaemia could be expected to survive three years. But looking at figures another way one can say that half the children with A.L.L. die within five years. Uncertainty is one of the hardest of all psychological burdens; in its outcome leukaemia is one of the most uncertain of all diseases.

Nowhere is the result of uncertainty more apparent than when parents discuss the problem of what to tell a child. (This dilemma is discussed elsewhere in this book, see Chapter 18.) For the child with leukaemia there is not a pressing need to explain details of the illness in order to gain his co-operation with treatment as there is with, say, cystic fibrosis. Of all conditions described in this book leukaemia has the most ominous ring to it, for many people imagine that it is always fatal. Much of the time while in remission the child seems to be quite normal. If there is a chance that he will stay in permanent remission then why bother him with the name? If he is going to die anyway why give him extra stress? As I have said earlier, each family must work out its own solution. In this particular context I will add only that I have not encountered a family who have reported distress in a child once he has been told; I have met many where the strain of secrecy was great.

WAYS OF HELPING CHILDREN AND FAMILIES

Once again, much of the discussion in Part One is relevant to ways of helping with psychological problems. To recapitulate the main points:

1. Parents should be given full information not only on their

child's condition but on what to expect. 'If only I had known she would be sleepy I would not have minded half as much, as it was I was worried out of my mind.'

2. Children should be given frequent opportunities to discuss their illness, from time to time with their doctor. It is easy to explain something to a six-year-old and then to forget to update information according to the child's age.

3. Whatever name one uses for the illness, it helps to develop a formula to use for neighbours, schoolmates and others who ask. One booklet of advice for parents recommends that neighbours are not told what the child is suffering from. If the child is not to know this is possibly a wise course of action, for neighbours' children have been known inadvertently to tell a child what is wrong with him. Against this is the undoubted fact that neighbours can provide welcome and readily available support, especially to a mother.

4. Psychological help can be offered in a number of ways. Some families will need none, others may at some time or another need and benefit from all. Ways that have been shown to be helpful are individual and group counselling for parents and for children both on an indefinite basis and for a limited time period. Whenever possible brothers and sisters should be considered as in need of help as well. A vital provision is that of ensuring that every family has at least one person they can contact when an immediate problem crops up.

5. Medical and nursing staff are not superhuman; they too need support from time to time and they need to have a back-up team to turn to in a crisis.

6. When a child has died, contact with school and hospital should not automatically and immediately stop.

The psychological problems caused by hair loss have not been discussed elsewhere in this book. The standard approach is to provide a wig and for some children this is effective in enabling them to return to school and to a normal life. But not all children agree to wear a wig, or to return to school at all until their hair has grown. I have been struck by the enormous variation from child to child. Some just say, 'call me Kojak' and sail apparently happily back into a full life. Others refuse even to leave hospital or house. I suspect that the child's expressed attitude owes much to the way his family have approached him and his illness, with the proviso that age has an additional effect, for all difficulties related to apearance are magnified in adolescence. Anticipation both of the loss and of the hair's return is of considerable value but there is no golden rule to apply to all children.

EDUCATION

The programme of treatment is such that children have many days off school. Given our present knowledge we are as yet uncertain of the effects on children's progress, although there are grounds for thinking that they may exist.

What is more certain is the need to provide children with as normal a life as possible and by sending them to an ordinary rather than a special school one is half way to achieving this end. Providing the child's doctor agrees, there is no reason why children should not take part in all school activities, including school trips. It is, of course, essential that teachers are made aware of the dangers from infection and that they be warned of possible side effects of treatment.

THE OUTLOOK

Medically the outlook improves continually. Now we are faced with a new problem: the leukaemic adult who may live a normal life span. This brings with it questions of marriage, fertility, and insurance risks. None has yet been answered but all are being asked.

23 Muscular dystrophy

Everyone has heard of leukaemia, and asthma, and most people can recognize a spastic. How many, though, are familiar with muscular dystrophy? How many parents, when first given the diagnosis, have any idea of the implications of the disease? In recent years the work of the Muscular Dystrophy Group has done much to help provide information but of all the conditions described in this book it remains one of the most taxing physically and psychologically, and one of the least understood by the general public.

DEFINITION

It is a progressive, usually inherited disease in which the muscles gradually waste away, the precise cause being unknown.

This is a simple definition but, as usual, the condition is not as simple as that. There are several types of muscular dystrophy, each with its own pattern of onset and development. Those described below are the ones that develop in childhood.

Duchenne

The most frequent and the most severe; it is rare that anyone with Duchenne type lives beyond their middle-twenties. Only boys are affected, but the mechanism of inheritance is such that females are carriers. (See page 164 for an explanation of the meaning of the word 'carrier'). The onset is usually apparent between the second and the fifth year.

Becker

This is rarer and milder than Duchenne, although the symptoms are similar. The onset comes in late childhood or early adulthood and it is often possible that a full working life can be led.

Once a boy has either Duchenne or Becker type muscular dystrophy parents often wonder about the possibility of subsequent boys having the same condition. This is not an easy question to answer and it is necessary to examine the family history plus the results of certain tests which have to be carried out on the mother. If it is established that the mother is the carrier there is a 50 per cent chance that subsequent boys will be affected.

Limb-girdle

Similar in pattern and severity to Becker, this type has a different inheritance pattern from the two already mentioned: either sex can be affected and if one child has it there is a one in four chance of siblings developing similarly.

FREQUENCY

This is a rare condition, approximately three boys in every 20,000 live births will have Duchenne, and that is by far the most common type.

CAUSES

Although the precise cause of muscle wasting is unknown, it is certain that in most cases the disease is inherited. In some there has been a mutation, a change in the genes which cannot be attributed to previous family factors.

THE PATTERN OF THE DISEASE

Duchenne is both the most common type and starts in the youngest age group and so will be delineated in some detail.

At first Duchenne boys seem to be quite normal but they are often late in walking. This in itself is not always a cause for great anxiety because a lot of children are late in some way or another and nine times out of ten mothers are told not to worry. In many cases there is no need for anxiety, although I do not think it is ever good advice just to say 'Don't worry' because in my experience this only increases the problem. It is better to explain to a mother why she should not worry about some things and to acknowledge, where appropriate, that other aspects of a child's health and development do warrant anxiety.

There remains the odd case when a child gets worse. He becomes increasingly clumsy, finds it more and more difficult to get up when he has fallen over and cannot manage stairs. The muscular wasting continues and by the age of about ten he is usually in a wheelchair, possibly with a somewhat curved spine. Gradually he loses the use of his arms. Sometimes his limbs stiffen into a sitting position which leads to discomfort in bed and it may be necessary to turn him several times a night.

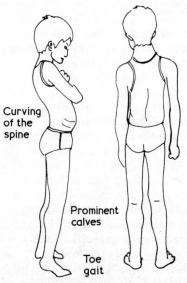

Curving
of the
spine

Prominent
calves

Toe
gait

Figure 8 Typical Duchenne posture

There are further complications, for the poor posture that comes from muscle weakness can affect respiratory functioning and this in turn means that children are more than usually prone to chest infections.

As if all this were not enough there is also a possible consequence of a lack of exercise: undue weight gain.

TREATMENT

There is no known cure for muscular dystrophy of any type.

MANAGEMENT

This is a different matter from treatment, for while no cure exists there is a great deal that can be done for the children, with the burden falling largely on the parents.

The general problems of parents, of children, and of their brothers and sisters are discussed in Chapters 2 and 18. In the rest of this section I touch upon some of the particular points that apply in this condition.

PSYCHOLOGICAL ASPECTS OF MANAGEMENT

Many parents of handicapped and sick children become accustomed to having their opinions dismissed. They are seen as fussy and overprotective. Sometimes this is fair comment. Overprotection is almost like a disease itself, a disease to which some parents are especially vulnerable. But because the onset of muscular dystrophy is relatively slow there is a greater than usual danger of parents not being taken seriously, of being told, as noted above, not to worry. In its early stages it is a difficult disease to diagnose and it is so rare that few GPs see more than one or two in a lifetime. The result of this combination of factors is that parents at first come to doubt their own competence, and then, once their fears have been shown to have some foundation, come to doubt the competence of doctors. The position is similar in many ways to that of parents of children with cystic fibrosis. One of the first psychological needs is to overcome both sets of doubts.

The immediate reaction pattern once a diagnosis has been given is discussed in Chapter 2. With parents of children with muscular dystrophy the realization that they can do something every day for their child is a provider of considerable psychological strength. It soon dawns on parents that whether they like it or not they are, in some ways, in a better position than doctors to maintain the quality of their child's life. As with similar situations, this is a mixed blessing, for it is easy to blame oneself when a child declines.

A less obvious psychological aid is the predictability of the course of the disease. By far the worst psychological aspects of some other diseases, for example lymphoblastic leukaemia, is the uncertainly about whether a child is likely to die this year, next year or whenever. At least the future for muscular dystrophy is well known.

We know lamentably little about the psychological factors operating on children. It is as well not to be misled by the brave face, amounting to bravado, that some boys manage to put on. I heard recently of a group of teenagers in a boarding school who laid bets on which of them would not return after the summer holidays. If work with other conditions, for example, spina bifida, is a guide, there is a great sea of uncharted worry which has to go somewhere.

When, as can happen, two brothers both have muscular dystrophy, the second learns from his observations of the older one's decline. This does not mean that no one needs explain anything to the second, he may be in the greater ignorance because of his half knowledge.

As a boy progressively loses skills, it is vital to try to assess which mean the most to him and to try to encourage him to maintain them if he possibly can. So if he does not mind being washed but hates being fed he should be allowed to go on managing for himself at mealtimes, no matter how messy he is.

The problems associated with a child facing death are discussed in Chapter 18.

PHYSICAL ASPECTS OF MANAGEMENT

Muscular dystrophy is essentially about movement; as the disease worsens, so movement is increasingly restricted. There are two main areas of physical help: what he does himself and what is done to his environment.

Exercise, physiotherapy, and the maintenance of a reasonable weight are all concerned with what he does himself. Swimming is particularly recommended but any regular exercise is to be encouraged. Physiotherapy can help to keep muscles in as good a working order as possible, but success depends not only on the technical skill of the therapist but also on the boy's willingness to co-operate. Weight gain is another area where parents and child must work together: it is tempting to give another cream cake to a boy in a wheelchair and it is tempting to ask for one.

Modifying the environment falls into two categories: the house and the wheelchair. For the parent the old saying 'Fore-warned is forearmed' comes into play and modifications to a house or flat, or moving altogether, must be kept in mind from the time of diagnosis. The permanent exhibition at the Disabled Living Foundation (see address list) gives some idea of ways in which a house can be adapted. One father told me that the best single piece of advice he can ever give is to buy a bungalow.

A wheelchair can bring with it a great mass of problems. It symbolizes another step downwards, it means that even more changes have to be made indoors and it seems to restrict movement more than ever.

In fact the picture is not as bleak as it appears and readers are advised to look at Philippa Russell's *The Wheelchair Child* (1978). There are two schools of thought on wheelchairs. The first says that children should be kept out of them for as long as possible and advocates the use of vigorous physiotherapy. The second, more popular in Britain, argues that a boy is really more mobile in a chair than he is tottering about on weak legs. And if he has got to be in a wheelchair sooner or later then the final acceptance is all the more humiliating if he has undergone a long and emotionally painful struggle to avoid an inevitable end. It is rather like adults growing old: we might as well do it gracefully.

EDUCATION

Most children with muscular dystrophy are able to attend ordinary nursery and then primary or pre-prep schools. Indeed, it is often at school that problems are first noticed. The child is a little clumsy, his handwriting is poor and he may have some difficulty with school work. At this stage the diagnosis can go terribly wrong. There is a current fashion in some educational circles to use an all embracing label, 'learning disability', for anyone who has problems with reading, writing, spelling, or maths. At first boys with muscular dystrophy seem to have many of the characteristics of learning disability and can be wrongly labelled. This sets parents and teachers off on a red herring trail which is of little value to anyone.

The picture is further confused by a generally reduced intelligence. On average there is an overall lowering of about twenty IQ points, so it is accurate to say that most boys fall into the low average range.

A special school must be considered once the muscles waste to an appreciable extent. There may be too many stairs in an ordinary school, or there may be no physiotherapy available. A case can also be made for the fact that special school teachers are better equipped than colleagues in ordinary education to cope with children facing death.

THE OUTLOOK

Children with muscular dystrophy can lead full and exciting lives, they can learn, they can pass some examinations, and they can make friends and enemies. But by sixteen most Duchenne boys are too handicapped to enter open employment and the outlook for them is not good. As the Warnock Report on Special Educational Needs put it, 'Provision for young people over sixteen with special educational needs has received little attention in the past . . . The field is relatively uncharted and is extremely complex . . .'

To pretend that the outlook for employment is otherwise does no service to parents or children. On the other hand change comes only in response to pressure and if those responsible for today's six-year-olds start exerting pressure now for improvements in post school facilities they may be achieved within ten years.

Muscular dystrophy

by Leslie A. Richardson
Headmaster of a special school

Coiled in your plastic shell
I look you over
For another sign.
Already private happenings
Need other people's help.

I speak with your mother
Of the future,
Of examinations,
Of jobs and holidays:
Well knowing the talk
Is academic.

Merciless time
Allows us to remember
The normalness of Spring
When the binoculars you held
Captured the sharp image
Of a bird.

Physiotherapy continues
For its own sake.

Your life moves quickly
Towards helplessness
So that I seem ageless
Having seen others.

Now is heaven;
Hell is the narrowing of movements
To a finger pointing;
An indication of intention
By a small nod.

Could I give you a year:
Put a brake on degeneration:
But your now is Now
And I shall speak brightly
Of the day
When the wheelchair
Tipped you into a hedge;
Well knowing the end of your future
Is within sight.

24   Renal failure

The kidneys lie one on each side of the spinal column. They are responsible for:

1. The elimination of waste materials containing nitrogen.
2. The maintenance of the water balance of the body.
3. The maintenance of the acid-based balance of the blood at a constant level.

Renal failure leads to the retention of waste products, anaemia and, ultimately, death.

A number of other physical problems are associated with renal failure in children: growth may fail, and in extreme cases dwarfism may occur; children may not mature sexually; bone abnormalities leading to rickets are not uncommon.

FREQUENCY

Kidney disease is common in children, especially in girls; by the age of five years one girl in 200 has some degree of kidney damage. Renal failure, leading to a need for a kidney machine and transplantation, is rare, affecting one or two children per million total population per year. In Britain this means that about ninety children aged five to fifteen years enter end-stage renal failure each year.

CAUSES

The major cause of chronic renal failure in infancy and early childhood is a congenital malformation of the kidney or urinary tract. In adolescence most problems are related to an acquired disease, the most common being glomerulonephritis, which follows an infection. The cause of this disease is not fully understood.

TREATMENT

Drug treatment can slow the progress of some forms of disease but if this fails it is essential to replace the kidney. The general aim with children is to effect a transplant, from a live donor or a cadaver, but there is a shortage of suitable kidneys. There is also no certainty that a transplant will be successful, at present rates there is about a 60 per cent chance that a child will remain fit for at least three years after the operation.

If the transplant is successful there can be a return to a relatively normal life. This statement must be taken literally, the key word being 'can be' and 'relatively,' for problems do not all end as the new kidney is introduced. The drugs needed to minimize the possibility of rejection also suppress the body's defence against infection, lead to the characteristic 'moon' face associated with steroid therapy, and stunt growth.

While waiting for a suitable kidney for transplantation the patient can be kept alive by dialysis, the use of an artificial kidney. The most common way of achieving this is by the use of haemodialysis, a kidney machine, which involves the insertion of large needles into a child's arm, sometimes via a permanently fixed shunt, enabling blood to flow through the machine, there to be processed as though by a kidney. This is a time-consuming procedure; three times a week for six or seven hours is not uncommon. It is also expensive, costing, in 1980, about £8,000 per year per patient.

An alternative technique used for some children is peritoneal dialysis, which uses the lining of the patient's own abdomen as an artificial kidney. This has an advantage over haemodyalisis in that it does not require expensive conversions to a home and the machine used requires less stringent supervision. On the other hand it usually involves five overnight sessions each week and is even more expensive than haemodyalisis.

An accompaniment to treatment is dietary restriction. There are essentially two types of diet for children in renal failure, one involving protein curtailment to keep waste products to a minimum, the other being low in salt, with a restriction on liquids.

PSYCHOLOGICAL FACTORS

The stress of looking after a child with a life-threatening

condition has been discussed in a general way in earlier chapters. There is no reason to believe that children in renal failure have a distinct and characteristic behaviour pattern but neither is there any doubt that this condition brings its own, colossal problems. No matter how much they try to avoid it, some parents begin to find the feelings of hostility they have towards the illness and its treatment extending to their child as well.

Some stress is directly and obviously related to the disease. Children tire easily, they cannot keep up with their friends in physical activities. Although some can attend full time school while on dialysis, a study published by Vass and colleagues in *The Lancet* in January 1977 noted that the average school attendance in the twenty-four children studied was 65 per cent. Dieting is a strain, and one boy has written, 'All the patients I know have in some way or other broken their diets.' (Andrew Northcote, writing in the third edition of the British Kidney Patient Association's *Silver Lining Appeal*.)

Some stress is directly and obviously related to the treatment. If a home is suitable for a machine parents are expected to devote an enormous amount of time to seeing that the treatment is carried out. If the home is not suitable the child will have to attend a hospital unit three times a week. If there is no portable machine available, holidays are likely to be severely curtailed.

At a psychologically deeper level children develop a distorted view of themselves and their body. At a time of growth when they would otherwise be learning with pride that their body is something over which they have increasing control they find not only that theirs is not growing as it should, it is malfunctioning to such an extent that they have to be hooked up to a machine. And if they swap the machine for a bit of someone else's body they will still not be exactly the same as everyone else. Ginette Raimbault studied sixty-nine children in Paris in 1973 and concluded, 'Whatever their behaviour and reactions, anxiety is a common, fundamental component of these children's psychological pattern . . . The body image is incomplete, empty . . . This may be related to one of the transplanted patients' major concerns, their sexual potency . . . Plans for the future practically never exist.' Other authors, some of whom contributed to Norman Levy's book *Living or Dying; Adaptation to Hemodialysis* (1974) argue that dependence and depression are two key results of treatment.

Not everyone would agree with such general conclusions. Barbara Korsch and colleagues in Los Angeles published a report in 1971 in which they pointed out that the stress associated with renal failure merely highlights patterns of behaviour that were present before. They go on to report that psychological states vary with the progress of the disease and its treatment. Drastic physical prodecures, with which the parents have to co-operate, can come so soon after the diagnosis that there is no time to adjust emotionally. As the treatment comes to be seen as successful so some parental feelings change and more warmth may be shown towards the child. A further stage, both medically and psychologically, is entered when a transplant is imminent. At first the operation is often invested 'only with hope and magic' but in time doubts set in and the Los Angeles report concludes that some of the most severe trials for patient, family and staff occur in the post-transplant period. They quote as an example the child who feels that he has to be well behaved to ensure that the transplanted kidney will function.

British work in this field has not entirely confirmed the American study, although direct comparisons cannot be made since there has not been an exact replication of the Los Angeles enquiry. Roy Howarth, who contributed to *The Lancet* paper already quoted, found that of the fourteen children who were disturbed at the beginning of the dialysis eleven were coping satisfactorily at the end of a year. In contrast, there was a tendency for parents to deteriorate during this period, although half of the twenty-four families coped well throughout.

THE OUTLOOK

About 96 per cent of patients below the age of fifteen years can now be expected to survive for at least four years, and possibly for much longer, under all forms of treatment. (About 100 children a year who could be treated with dialysis or transplants are dying in Britain because of a shortage of facilities.)

The outlook for survivors can be bright but the ambivalence of the picture is summed up in two quotations from the *Silver Lining Appeal*. Andrew Timms, writing in the fourth edition, ended his article, 'In retrospect, once transplanted I have never looked back ... I now look forward to a future hopefully untainted by the problems of ill health.' Timothy Ward, in the fifth edition, wrote:

> *The difference of machine and graft*
> *Is really very small*
> *The worry's just a different kind*
> *That's if it works at all.*

25 Spina bifida and hydrocephalus

Spina bifida is the commonest major abnormality present at birth. It was described 2,000 years ago and yet it remains one of the hidden conditions: many people have come across the name but few know exactly what it is. Even parents of a spina bifida child are often strangely ignorant. This is partly because children with severe forms of the condition used to die within a few weeks of birth; it is partly because there are several different forms, each with its own outcome.

DEFINITIONS

Bifid is from a Latin word meaning split. A child with spina bifida is born with some of the bones in the spine not properly joined together, leaving a split through which the spinal cord protrudes. This sounds very unpleasant and in some cases it looks very unpleasant before it is treated. But, as cannot be said too often, not all spina bifida is the same.

Spina bifida occulta generally results in little more obvious than a slight swelling on the back, or possibly other slight indications; the child's functioning is usually quite normal.

Spina bifida aperta (sometimes called *spina bifida cystica*) is the condition in which some of the spinal cord protrudes through the split into a sac filled with fluid. In turn this type is divided into two forms:

1. *meningocele*: the spinal cord remains intact and in its correct position, only its covering protrudes, usually covered with skin. The child can function within normal limits.

2. *myelemeningocele*: this is by far the most serious type, in which the cord itself protrudes into a sac, with consequent

neurological impairment. But there are differences even within this category, with the nature of the resulting handicap depending on the site and extent of the defect.

The effects of myelemeningocele can include: paralysis and deformities of the lower limbs, and sometimes of the upper, skin insensitivity, incontinence, kidney infections, and impaired intelligence. This a formidable list; the parent of a severely affected child has a heavy burden.

Hydrocephalus is an associated condition. Literally it means water in the head and is caused by a build up of excess fluid within the brain. If untreated it leads to an enlarged head and possibly serious malfunctioning of the brain.

Hydrocephalus can occur independently of spina bifida and not all spina bifida children have hydrocephalus. When they do, and this is the case in up to 90 per cent of myelemeningoceles, the child's problems are, of course, increased significantly. On its own it can result in uneven intellectual development and some paralysis.

FREQUENCY

Spina bifida: about five in every 2,000 live births. Hydrocephalus: about 1.2 in every 2,000 live births.

These figures pertain to 1977; with increased use of screening procedures it is likely that they will fall.

An unexplained finding is the regional differences in the distribution of spina bifida: it is most common in Ireland, Wales, Scotland, and the North of England and least common in East Anglia and the South of England. Various theories have been put forward but none has yet been shown to be true.

CAUSES

Spina bifida and hydrocephalus result from congenital abnormalities, i.e. abnormalities present at conception or early in pregnancy. Beyond that little is known. Research has shown nothing conclusive about the possible causal effect of parents' age, diet, or environmental conditions, and there is now an assumption that there is unlikely to be one single cause. Parents with a spina bifida child are advised to seek genetic counselling if they are considering having another child.

TREATMENT

Spina bifida is irreversible and there is no cure. Modern surgery has so developed, though, that the spine can now be covered to prevent infection and life can be prolonged.

The outlook for children with hydrocephalus changed dramatically in 1958 when a shunt was inserted into a child's head and fluid was drained off artificially. 'Valve' and 'shunt' are often used as though they meant the same thing; in fact shunt refers to the whole apparatus, valve to a part of it. Two forms of valve are in current use. One of them, the Spitz-Holter, is the joint invention of a surgeon and an engineer, the latter of whom had a child with hydrocephalus.

Once the initial surgery has been undertaken and the condition stabilized, treatment aims at making the most of the child's strengths, alleviating, as far as possible, the results of the damage already done. Physiotherapy is likely to be a central part of many children's lives and a variety of physical aids can be called into play, from a wheelchair to a urinary device. On the other hand none of these may be necessary; it is impossible to generalize.

MANAGEMENT AT HOME

An early question from most parents relates to the way in which their child will develop. In the last thirty years a body of knowledge has increased so that we can now make broad but fairly reliable predictions about the extent of impairment to be expected. Children with a shunt, for example, are usually less intelligent than those who do not need one. Spina bifida with hydrocephalus usually leads to lowered intelligence; without hydrocephalus the range of intelligence is closer to the normal. (This is not to say that all such children will be of normal intelligence, it is the *range* that is normal.)

The primary need, then, is to establish the nature and extent of the damage and from this to consider the course that other children have followed. What follows is a general description of what can occur.

IMPAIRED MOVEMENT

Many children have some degree of impairment in their legs,

some being unable to walk at all. Next to incontinence, immobility is often reported by parents to be the most wearing aspect of spina bifida, especially as the child becomes older and heavier. I know one mother who is normally placid and cheerful. The only time I have seen her upset was when she described the near impossibility of travelling by bus with two young children, one of whom is unable to walk.

Many children also grow up unable to use their hands perfectly. This poor hand use may be due to the original condition, it may be due to lack of practice. A child who cannot crawl and toddle does not get a chance to practise handling objects as does his non-handicapped brother. If a child cannot move himself to things, things should be brought to him.

LANGUAGE

A common characteristic of spina bifida and hydrocephalic children is the ready picking up of words without the corresponding skill of verbal reasoning. Children can repeat phrases but have difficulty in giving an account of an event in their own words. The result is a ready chatter which seems bright superficially, and is known as the Cocktail Party Syndrome. Some people are misled by this characteristic into thinking that a wide vocabulary means high intelligence. I knew one father who took his child half way round the world, seeking one psychological opinion after another, because he just could not believe that his daughter was unable to understand the words that came so readily and attractively from her tongue.

SKIN INSENSITIVITY

Some children suffer from a degree of skin insensitivity, i.e. they do not have the same capacity to feel pain as others. The main potential dangers here are heat and minor cuts. A child can sit far too close to a fire and get quite badly burned without feeling anything. Children must be taught to examine their skin regularly so that minor abrasions can be attended to before they become infected.

INCONTINENCE

The essential problem is a failure of the nervous system to successfully transmit to the brain an indication of a need to go to the lavatory. In mild cases urine can be expressed regularly by pressure from the hands on the lower part of the abdomen and some children learn to do this themselves. In some more serious cases children have urinary diversions, and in some cases a boy may have to wear a penile bag and a girl incontinence pads (over which normal clothing can be worn). As children grow up urinary difficulties produce some of the mose severe psychological problems.

MANAGEMENT AT SCHOOL

A recent London survey showed that 40 per cent of a group of children with spina bifida were attending ordinary schools, often receiving extra help only with toiletting (See *The Child with Spina Bifida* by Elizabeth Anderson and Bernie Spain). If an ordinary school is not thought to be the best place the usual alternatives are a special school for the physically handicapped or for the slow learning.

The outstanding educational characteristic is the uneven nature of most children's performance. The mechanics of reading, for example, may present no problem whereas mathematics does. Skill in maths is related to skill at organizing one's world in space. This is probably why so many good chess players are also good at maths. One consistent result produced by educational investigations of children with spina bifida is that their spatial skills are not good and they find jigsaws, and anything else to do with two-dimensional patterns, very hard. They rarely shine at maths.

In common with other neurologically impaired children they face two other educational drawbacks: distractibility and poor handwriting. They are easily diverted from the task in hand, and teachers and parents often complain, 'If only he could concentrate he could do so much better'. This is, no doubt, true, but it is rather like saying, 'If only he were not handicapped he could run 100 metres.'

Handwriting may seem a minor difficulty compared to penile bags and wheelchairs, yet it can be a constant source of niggling frustration to a child, and poor handwriting can be improved with careful teaching. Anyone interested in following this up should contact the Association for Spina Bifida and Hydrocephalus (see address list). For references to educational research see D. Pilling's *The Child with Spina Bifida* (1973).

DANGER SIGNS

It is essential that anyone looking after a child with a shunt is aware of the indications that something is wrong. The possible dangers and the signs associated with them are:

A blocked valve: headaches, vomiting, drowsiness, possibly a fit.

Infection of a shunt: fever, night sweating, vomiting, possibly poor appetite, irritability.

A disconnected shunt: a lump behind the ear or swelling along the length of the tube.

If any of these is suspected medical advice should be sought immediately.

THE OUTLOOK

The long-term outlook is hard to predict for it is only in the last twenty years or so that many children have been able to live to adulthood. Prospects for employment can, to some extent, be judged from the child's ability to cope with educational demands. If he has been able to manage in an ordinary school there is every possibility of his holding down a job in open employment. If he has been to a special school there may still be the possibility of employment but everything will depend on the extent of the handicap.

We do, however, know something of the outlook facing adolescents, thanks to the work of the psychologist Steven Dorner. Many seem to be remarkably ignorant of their condition, possibly reflecting their parents' lack of understanding. Boys seem to be more adversely affected than girls by urinary appliances and there is a high degree of social isolation in both sexes. It seems likely that this isolation is not due to which type of school was attended, rather it is dependent on the young person's mobility. Assistance in developing independence is a high priority for the sixteen-plus age group.

Part Four

References

ANDERSON, ELIZABETH and SPAIN, BERNIE (1977) *The Child with Spina Bifida*. London: Methuen.

ANTHONY, SYLVIA (1971) *The Discovery of Death in Childhood and After*. London: Allen Lane.

ATKIN, MARGARET, (1974) The doomed family: observations on the lives of parents and children facing repeated mortality. In L. Burton (ed.) *The Care of the Child Facing Death*. London: Routledge & Kegan Paul.

BEE, HELEN (1978) *The Developing Child*. New York: Harper & Row.

BLACK, DORA and STURGE, CLAIRE (1979) The young child and his siblings. In J. Howells (ed.) Modern Perspectives in the Psychology of Infancy. New York: Bruner Mazel.

BLUEBOND-LANGNER, MYRA (1978) *The Private Worlds of Dying Children*. Princeton, N.J.: Princeton University Press.

BOSWELL, D.M. and WINGROVE, J.M. (1974) *The Handicapped Person in the Community*. London: Tavistock Publications.

BOWLBY, JOHN (1951) *Child Care and the Growth of Love*. Harmondsworth: Penguin Books.

BOWLBY, JOHN (1969) *Attachment and Loss: 1 Attachment*. London: Hogarth Press.

BURTON, LINDY (ed.) (1974) *The Care of the Child Facing Death*. London: Routledge & Kegan Paul.

_____ (1975) *The Family Life of Sick Children*. London: Routledge & Kegan Paul.

CARR, JANET (1970) Handicapped children: counselling the parents. *Devel.Med. & Child Neurol.* 12: 230.

CASSELL, S. and PAUL, M.H. (1967) The role of puppet therapy on the environmental responses of children hospitalized for cardiac catheterization. *Journal of Pediatrics* 71: 233.

CLARKE, A.M. and A.D.B. (eds) (1976) *Early Experience: Myth and Evidence*. Shepton Mallet: Open Books.

_____ (1978) *Readings from Mental Deficiency*. London: Methuen.

COBB, H.V. (1972) *The Forecast of Fulfilment*. New York: Teachers College Press.

COPELAND, JAMES (1973) *For the Love of Ann*. London: Arrow Books.

CRAFT, MICHAEL and CRAFT, ANN (1978) *Sex and the Mentally Handicapped*. London: Routledge & Kegan Paul.

CRAFT, MICHAEL (1979) *Tredgold's Mental Retardation*. London: Bailliere Tindall.

DAVIE, R., BUTLER, N., and GOLDSTEIN, H. (1972) *From Birth to Seven*. London: Longman.

DEPARTMENT OF EDUCATION AND SCIENCE (1964) *Statistics of Education 1963*. London: HMSO.

DEPARTMENT OF EDUCATION AND SCIENCE (1972) *The Education of the Visually Handicapped* (The Vernon Report). London: HMSO.

DEPARTMENT OF EDUCATION AND SCIENCE (1978) *Special Educational Needs* (The Warnock Report). London: HMSO.

DEPARTMENT OF HEALTH AND SOCIAL SECURITY (1976) *Fit for the Future* (The Court Report). London: HMSO.

DEPARTMENT OF HEALTH AND SOCIAL SECURITY (1976) *Report of the Expert Group on Play for Children in Hospital*. London: HMSO.

DINNAGE, ROSEMARY (1972) *The Handicapped Child: Research Review*, Vol.II. London: Longman.

DISABILITY ALLIANCE (1979) *The Disability Rights Handbook*.

DONALDSON, MARGARET (1978) *Children's Minds*. London: Collins/Fontana.

DORNER, STEVEN (1977) Sexual interest and activity in adolescents with spina bifida. *J. Child Psychol. & Psychiat*. 18: 229.

DOUGLAS, J.W.B. (1975) Early hospital admissions and later disturbances in behaviour and learning. *Devel. Med. & Child Neurol*. 17: 456.

EDELSTON, H. (1943) Separation anxiety in young children: a study of hospital cases. *Genetic Psychol. Monog*. 28: 3.

FAGIN, C.M. (1964) The case for rooming in when young children are hospitalized. *Nurs. Sci*. 2: 324.

FOLSTEIN, S. and RUTTER, M. (1977) Infantile autism: a genetic study of 21 twin pairs. *J. Child Psychol. & Psychiat*. 18: 297.

GALLOWAY, DAVID (1976) *Case Studies in Classroom Management*. London: Longman.

GELLERT, E. (1956) Reducing the emotional stress of hospitalization for children. *Am. J. Occup. Therapy* 12: 125.

GOFFMAN, ERVING (1963) *Stigma*. Harmondsworth: Penguin Books.

GREEN, LEN (1969) Comparison of school attainments. *Special Education* 58: 9.

GREENGROSS, WENDY (1976) *Entitled to Love*. National Marriage Guidance Council.

GREGORY, SUSAN (1976) *The Deaf Child and his Family*. London: Allen & Unwin.

HARRIS, P. (1979) Children, their parents and hospital. Unpublished Ph.D. thesis, University of Nottingham.

HARVEY, SUSAN and HALES-TOOKE, ANN (eds) (1972) *Play in Hospital*. London: Faber & Faber.

HEWETT, SHEILA (1970) *The Family and the Handicapped Child.* London: Allen & Unwin.

JACKSON, J., BOOTH, M., and HARRIS, B. (1977) *Clarke Hall and Morrison's Law Relating to Children and Young Persons.* London: Butterworth.

JOHNSON, J.C. (1962) *Educating Hearing Impaired Children in Ordinary Schools.* Manchester: Manchester University Press.

JOLLY, JUNE (1969) Play is work. *The Lancet* 2: 487.

KEW, STEPHEN (1975) *Handicap and Family Crisis.* London: Pitman.

KORSCH, B., FINE, R., GRUSHKIN, C. and NEGRETE, V. (1971) Experiences with children and their families during extended hemodialysis and kidney transplantation. *Pediatric Clinics of North Am.* 18: 625.

LEVY, N. (ed.) (1974) *Living or Dying: Adaptation to Hemodyalisis.* Springfield, Ill.: C.C. Thomas.

LINDHEIM, R., GLASER, H.H. and COFFIN, C. (1972) *Changing Hospital Environments for Children.* Boston: Harvard University Press.

LINDUSKA, N. (1947) *My Polio Past.* Pellegrini & Cudahy.

MAC KEITH, R. (1973) The feelings and behaviour of parents of handicapped children. *Devel. Med. & Child Neurol.* 15: 24.

MATTINSON, J.M. (1975) *Marriage and Mental Health.* London: Institute of Marital Studies, Tavistock Institute of Human Relations.

MILLAR, SUSANNA (1968) *The Psychology of Play.* Harmondsworth: Penguin Books.

MINISTRY OF HEALTH (1959) *Report of the Committee on the Welfare of Children in Hospital* (The Platt Report). London: HMSO.

NOLAND, ROBERT L. (1970) *Counselling Parents of the Mentally Retarded.* Springfield, Ill.: C.C. Thomas.

PARK, CLARA (1967) *The Siege.* London: Colin Smythe.

PEINE, HERMANN and HOWARTH, ROY (1975) *Children and Parents.* Harmondsworth: Penguin Books.

PILLING, D. (1973) *The Child with Cerebral Palsy.* Slough: N.F.E.R.

_____ (1973) *The Child with Spina Bifida.* Slough: N.F.E.R.

_____ (1973) *The Handicapped Child: Research Review III.* London: Longman.

PRUGH, D.G., STAUB, E.M., SANDS, H.H., KIRSCHBAUM, R.N., and LENIHAN, G.A. (1953) A study of the emotional reactions of children and families to hospitalization and illness. *Am. J. of Orthopsychiat.* 23:70.

RAIMBAULT, GINETTE (1973) Psychological aspects of chronic renal failure. *Nephron* 11: 252.

RICHARDSON, S.A. (1971) Handicap, appearance and stigma *Soc. Sci. & Med.* 5: 621.

ROBERTSON, JAMES and BOWLBY, JOHN (1952) Reponses of young children to separation from their mothers. *Courier: Revue Médico-Sociale de l'Enfance* (Centre International de l'Enfance) 2:131.

ROBERTSON, JAMES (1970) *Young Children in Hospital*. London: Tavistock Publications.

ROITH, A.I. (1963) The myth of parental attitudes. *Brit. Jnl of Mental Subnormality* 9: 51.

RUSSELL, PHILIPPA (1978) *The Wheelchair Child*. London: Souvenir Press.

RUTTER, MICHAEL, TIZARD, JACK, and WHITMORE, KINGSLEY (1970) *Education, Health and Behaviour*. London: Longman.

RUTTER, MICHAEL (1972) *Maternal Deprivation Reassessed*. Harmondsworth: Penguin Books.

RUTTER, MICHAEL and HERSOV, LIONEL (1976) *Child Psychiatry: Modern Approaches*. Oxford: Blackwell.

SAMEROFF, A.J. and CHANDLER, M.J. (1975) Reproductive risks and the continuum of caretaking casualty. In F.D. Horowitz *et al.* (eds) *Review of Childhood Development Research* 4: 187.

SAUNDERS, CECILY (1969) The management of fatal illness in childhood. *Proc. Roy. Soc. Med.* 62: 550.

SCHIFF, HARRIET (1979) *The Bereaved Parent*. London: Souvenir Press.

SCOTT, ROBERT (1970) The construction of conceptions of stigma by professional experts. In J. Douglas (ed.) *Deviance and Respectability*. New York: Basic Books.

SELFE, LORNA and NEWSON, ELIZABETH (1977) *Nadia*. London: Academic Press.

SHENNAN, VICTORIA (1977) *Help Your Child Understand Sex*. London: Nat. Soc. for Ment. Hand. Children.

SKYNNER, A.C.R. (1976) *One Flesh, Separate Persons*. London: Constable.

SOBOL, HARRIET LANGSAM (1978) *My Brother Stephen is Retarded*. London: Gollancz.

STACEY, M., DEARDEN, R., PILL, R. and ROBINSON, D. (1970) *Hospitals, Children and their Families*. London: Routledge & Kegan Paul.

SWINY, C. (1975) Follow-up study of 900 patients with cerebral palsy. Paper presented at the Annual Meeting of the American Academy for Cerebral Palsy.

TINDALL, GILLIAN (1965) *A Handbook on Witches*. London: Arthur Barker.

TIZARD, BARBARA and HARVEY, DAVID (1977) *Biology of Play*. London: Heinemann.

TIZARD, JACK (1964) *Community Services for the Mentally Handicapped*. Oxford: Oxford University Press.

TIZARD, JACK and GRAD, J.G. (1961) *The Mentally Handicapped and their Families*. Maudsley Monog. 7. Oxford: Oxford University Press.

TURK, J. (1964) Impact of cystic fibrosis on family functioning. *Pediatrics* 34:67.

VASS, V.J. AND THE LONDON CHILDREN'S HOME DIALYSIS GROUP (1977) Home Dialysis in children. *The Lancet* 1: 243;

VAUGHAN, G.F. (1957) Children in Hospital. *The Lancet* 2: 1117.

VERNON, D.T.A., FOLEY, J.M., SIPOWICZ, R.R., and SCHULMAN J.L. (1965) *The Psychological Responses of Children to Hospitalization and Illness.* Springfield, Ill.: C.C. Thomas.

VERNON, D.T.A., SCHULMAN, J.L. and FOLEY, J.M. (1966) Changes in children's behaviour after hospitalization. *J. Diseases of Children* 3: 581.

VERNON, P.E. (1979) *Intelligence, Heredity and Environment.* San Francisco: W.H. Freeman.

VINSTAINER, M.A. and WOLFER, J.A. (1975) Psychological preparation for surgical patients: the effect on children's and parents' stress responses and adjustment. *Pediatrics* 56: 187.

VOLUNTARY COUNCIL FOR HANDICAPPED CHILDREN (1978) *Help Starts Here.*

WING, LORNA (ed.) (1976) *Early Childhood Autism.* Oxford: Pergamon.

WOODWARD, J. and JACKSON, D. (1968) Educational reactions in burned children and their mothers. *Br. J. Plastic Surgery.* 13: 316.

WORTHINGTON, ANN *In Touch.* Distributed from 10 Norman Road, Sale, Cheshire.

YUDKIN, SIMON (1967) Children and death. *The Lancet* 7: 37.

Further reading

1. FOR ADULTS

Apart from the books and articles mentioned in the reference list the following are recommended for further reading.

ANDERSON, ELIZABETH and SPAIN, BERNIE (1977) *The Child with Spina Bifida*. London: Methuen.

ANTHONY, E.J. and KOUPERNIK, C. (1973) *International Yearbook for Child Psychiatry and Allied Disciplines*. New York: Wiley.

BLECK, EUGENE E. and NAGEL, DONALD A. (1975) *Physically Handicapped Children: A Medical Atlas for Teachers*. London: Grune & Stratton.

BLENCOE, SUSAN (1969) *Cerebral Palsy and the Young Child*. Edinburgh: E. & S. Livingstone.

FINNIE, NANCIE (1968) *Handling the Young Cerebral Palsied Child at Home*. London: Heinemann.

FRAIBERG, SELMA (1978) *Insights from the Blind*. London: Souvenir Press.

FREEMAN, PEGGY (1975) *Understanding the Deaf Blind Child*. London: Heinemann.

LAGOS, JORGE C. (1974) *Help for the Epileptic Child*. London: Macdonald & Jane's.

NATIONAL CHILDREN'S BUREAU *Highlight* series. This is a series of information sheets summarizing recent research.

RICHARDSON, ROSAMOND (ed.) (1980) *Losses: Talking about Bereavement*. Shepton Mallet: Open Books.

SCOTT, EILEEN P., JAN, JAMES E., and FREEMAN, ROGER D. (1977) *Can't Your Child See?* Baltimore: University Park Press.

STONE, JUDITH and TAYLOR, FELICITY (1977) *A Handbook for Parents with a Handicapped Child*. London: Arrow Books.

WRIGHT, DAVID (1969) *Deafness: A Personal Account*. London: Allen Lane.

2. FOR CHILDREN

a) On handicap

Harriet Langsam Sobol's book has been mentioned in the references to the main text. Others are:

ANON (undated) *Rupert and his Friends*. Slough: Ames Company.
FANSHAWE, E. (1975) *Rachel*. London: Bodley Head. (Physical handicap).
JESSEL, C. (1975) *Mark's Wheelchair Adventures*. London: Methuen.
LARSEN, H. (1976) *Don't Forget Tom*. London: A. & C. Black. (Mental handicap).
PETER, D. (1976) *Claire and Emma*. London: A. & C. Black. (Hearing loss).
PETERSEN, P. (1976) *Sally Can't See*. London: A. & C. Black.

b) For children about to go into hospital

ADAMSON, J and ADAMSON, G. (1971) *Topsy and Tim go to Hospital*. Glasgow: Blackie.
BEMELMANS, L. (1957) *Madeline*. London: Andre Deutsch.
COPPARD, A. (1978) *Get Well Soon*. London: Heinemann.
JESSEL, C. and JOLLY, H. (1972) *Paul in Hospital*. London: Methuen.
JONES, A. (1969) *Dan Berry Goes to Hospital*. Glasgow: Blackie.
REY, M. and REY, H. (1967) *Zozo Goes to Hospital*. London: Chatto & Windus.
WEBER, A. (1970) *Liza Goes to Hospital*. Glasgow: Blackie.

Address list

1. National associations concerned with particular groups

Association for All Speech-Impaired Children (AFASIC), 347 Central Markets, Smithfield, London EC1A 9NH. (01-236 3632)

Association to Combat Huntington's Chorea, Nansen House, 64 Millbank, London SW1. (01-834 6326)

Association of Parents of Vaccine-Damaged Children, 2 Church Street, Shipston-on-Stour, Warwicks. CV36 4AP.

Association for Research into Restricted Growth, 2 Mount Court, 81 Central Hill, London SE19 1BS

Association for Spina Bifida and Hydrocephalus, Tavistock House North, Tavistock Square, London WC1H 9HJ. (01-388 1382)

British Deaf Association, 38 Victoria Place, Carlisle CA1 1HU (0228 20188) Mainly concerned with adults; some publications relevant to children.

British Diabetic Association, 3-4 Alfred Place, London WC1E 7EE. (01-636 7355)

British Epilepsy Association, 3-6 Alfred Place, London WC1E 7EE. (01-580 2704)

British Heart Foundation, 57 Gloucester Place, London W1H 4DH. (01-935 0185)

British Kidney Patient Association, Bordon, Hants. (042 03 2021)

Brittle Bone Society, 63 Byron Crescent, Dundee DD3 6SS. (0382 87130)

Chest and Heart Association, Tavistock House North, Tavistock Square, London WC1H 9HJ. (01-387 3012)

Cleft Lip and Palate Association, Dental Dept, The Hospital for Sick Children, Great Ormond Street, London WC1N 3JH. (01-405 9200)

Colostomy Welfare Group, 38 Eccleston Square, London SW1U 1PB. (01-828 5175)

Cystic Fibrosis Research Trust, 5 Blyth Road, Bromley, Kent BR1 3RS. (01-461 7211)

Down's Children's Association, Quinbourne Community Centre, Ridgacre Road, Birmingham B32 2TW. (021-427 1374)

Friedreich's Ataxia Group, Bolsover House, 5-6 Clipstone Street, London W1. (01-636 2042)

Haemophilia Society, PO Box 9, 16 Trinity Street, London SE1 1DE. (01-407 1010)

Lady Hoare Trust for Physically Disabled Children, 7 North Street, Midhurst, W. Sussex GU29 9DJ. (073-081 3696)

Leukaemia Research Fund, 61 Great Ormond Street, London WC1. (01-405 9200)

Leukaemia Society, 28 Eastern Road, London N2. (01-883 4703)

MIND (National Association for Mental Health), 22 Harley Street, London W1N 2ED. (01-637 0741) Concerned with the legal rights of the mentally ill and handicapped. It has an information service and a range of publications.

Multiple Sclerosis Society, 4 Tachbrook Street, London SW14 1SJ. (01-834 8231)

Muscular Dystrophy Group of Great Britain, Nattrass House, 35 Macaulay Road, London SW4 OQP. (01-720 8055)

National Association for Deaf/Blind and Rubella Handicapped, 164 Cromwell Lane, Coventry CV4 8AP, Warwicks. (0203 462579)

National Association for the Education of the Partially Sighted, Joseph Clark School, Vincent Road, Higham Park, London E4. (01-527 8818)

National Association for Mental Handicap, 5 Fitzwilliam Place, Dublin. ((Dublin) 76 6035)

National Deaf Children's Society, 31 Gloucester Place, London W1H 4EA. (01-486 3251)

National Eczema Society, Mary Ward House, 5-7 Tavistock Place, London WC1. (01-387 9681)

National Elfrida Rathbone Society, 83 Mosley Street, Manchester M2 3QG. (061 236 5358) National organization concerned particularly with the ESN(M). Holiday play-schemes, literacy classes, etc. making particular use of volunteers. Research projects also carried out with particular interest in vocational training and employment.

National Society for Autistic Children, 1a Golders Green Road, London NW11. (01-453 4375)

National Society for Mentally Handicapped Children, 117 Golden Lane, London EC1Y ORT. (01-253 9433)

National Society of Phenylketonuria and Allied Disorders, 6 Rawdon Close, Palace Fields, Runcorn, Cheshire. (092 85 65081)

Royal National Institute for the Blind, 224 Great Portland Street, London W1N 6AA. (01-388 1266)

Royal National Institute for the Deaf, 105 Gower Street, London WC1E 6BR. (01-387 8033)

Scottish Council for Spastics, 22 Corstorphine Road, Edinburgh. (031-337 2804)

Scottish Society for the Mentally Handicapped, 69 West Regent Street, Glasgow G2 2AN. (041-331 1551)

Scottish Spina Bifida Association, 190 Queensferry Road, Edinburgh. (031-332 0743)

Spastics Society, 12 Park Crescent, London W1N 4EQ. (01-636 5020)

2. General

Association of Professions for the Mentally Handicapped, King's Fund Centre, 126 Albert Street, London NW1 7NF. (01-267 6111) For all, including parents, concerned with the improvement of services.

Breakthrough, A. Kenyon, 103 Ridgeway Drive, Bromley, Kent. (01-857 4170) Arranges family holidays for deaf and multi-handicapped deaf children. Other activities also.

British Council for the Rehabilitation of the Disabled, Tavistock House South, Tavistock Square, London WC1 9LB. (01-387 4037)

British Sports Association for the Disabled, Stoke Mandeville Stadium, Harvey Road, Aylesbury, Bucks. HP21 8PP. (0296 84848)

Central Bureau for Educational Visits and Exchanges, 43 Dorset Street, London W1H 3FN (01-486 5101) 3 Bruntsfield Crescent, Edinburgh EH10 4HD. (031-447 8024)

Centre on Environment for the Handicapped, 126 Albert Street, London NW1 7NF. (01-267 6111)

Child Poverty Action Group, 1 Macklin Street, London WC1. (01-242 9149)

Community Service Volunteers, 237 Pentonville Road, London N1. (01-278 6601)

Contact a Family Project, Francis House, Francis Street, London SW1P 1DE. (01-828 7364) Aims to give families with a handicapped child living at home contact with other families in the same situation and area.

Council for Children's Welfare, 183-189 Finchley Road, London NW3. (01-624 8766)

Department of Health and Social Security (Information Division), Alexander Fleming House, Elephant and Castle, London SE1. (01-407 5522)

Disability Alliance, 96 Portland Place, London W1N 4EX. (01-794 1536)

Disabled Campers' Club, 28 Coote Road, Bexleyheath, Kent.

Disabled Living Foundation, 356 Kensington High Street, London W14 8NS. (01-602 2491) Information and advice on house design and aids for the handicapped.

Family Fund, Beverley House, Shipton Road, York YO3 6RB. (0904 29241)

Family Planning Association, 27-35 Mortimer Street, London W1N 7RJ. (01-636 7866)

Foundation for the Study of Infant Deaths, 23 St Peter's Square, London W6 9NW. (01-235 1721) (out of office hours 01-748 7768)

Fund for the Training of Handicapped Children in Arts and Crafts, 94 Claremont Road, Wallasey, Merseyside L45 6UE.

Handicapped Adventure Playground Association, Fulham Palace, Bishop's Avenue, London SW6 6EA (01-736 4443)

Handicapped Education and Aid Research Unit, City of London Polytechnic, Walburgh House, Bigland Street, London EC1. Advice and help with making special furniture and aids for the handicapped.

Home Library, J. Wheeler, 23 Canning Street, Brighton BN2 2EF. Non-profit making concern which provides simple-language versions of popular picture books for children.

In Touch, Ann Worthington, 10 Norman Road, Sale, Cheshire M33 3DF. (061-962 4441) A circular to enable parents, mainly of the mentally handicapped, share information.

Institute for Mental Subnormality, Wolverhampton Road, Kidderminster, Worcestershire. (0562 850251) Offers full training programme, publications, workshops etc. for everyone involved with the mentally handicapped, including parents and teachers. Particularly useful for information on teaching techniques, including behaviour modification and use of workshops.

Institute for Research into Multiple and Mental Handicap, 16 Fitzroy Square, London W1P 5HQ. (01-387 9571)

Invalid Children's Aid Association, 126 Buckingham Palace Road, London SW1. (01-730 9891)

John Tracy Clinic, 806 West Adams Boulevard, Los Angeles, California 90007, USA. Offers among other things a correspondence course for parents of deaf children.

KIDS National Centre for Cued Speech, 17 Sedlescombe Road, London SW6 7RE. (01-381 0335)

Kith and Kids, 6 Grosvenor Road, London N10. (01-883 8762) Family group projects for all categories of handicapped children and their families.

London College of Furniture, 41 Commercial Road, London EC1. (01-247 1953) Play equipment and toy design course.

Medic-Alert Foundation, 9 Hanover Street, London W1. (01-499 2261)

National Association for One Parent Families, 255 Kentish Town Road, London NW5 2LX.

National Association of Swimming Clubs for the Handicapped, 4 Hillside Gardens, Northwood, Middlesex. (65 27784)

National Association for the Welfare of Children in Hospital, 7 Exton Street, London SE1 8VE. (01-261 1738)

National Bureau for Handicapped Students, Thomas Coram Foundation, 40 Brunswick Square, London WC1. (01-278 3127) To meet the needs of handicapped students interested in further or higher education. Information on grants, courses etc.

National Childminding Association, Camrie Bastred, Westerham, Kent. (51 63465) (Send SAE)

National Children's Bureau, 8 Wakley Street, Islington, EC1V 7QE. (01-278 9441) A wide range of publications; library; information service.

National Council for Special Education, 1 Wood Street, Stratford-upon-Avon CV37 6JE. (0789 5332)

National Fund for Research into Crippling Diseases, Vincent House, 1a Springfield Road, Horsham, Sussex. (0403 64101)

National Marriage Guidance Council, 76a New Cavendish Street, London W1. (01-580 1087)

Network, Bedford House, 35 Emerald Street, WC1. (01-504 3001)

Ombudsman, Church House, Great Smith Street, London SW1.

Parents for Children, 222 Camden High Street, London NW1. (01-485 7548) An adoption agency specializing in handicapped children.

Photography for the Disabled, 190 Secrett House, Ham Close, Ham, Richmond, Surrey.

Pre-school Playgroups Association, Alford House, Aveline Street, London SE11 5DJ. (01-582 8871)

Riding for the Disabled Association, c/o British Horse Society, National Equestrian Centre, Stoneleigh, Kenilworth, Warwicks. (0203 56107)

Joseph Rowntree Memorial Trust, The Secretary, The Family Fund, PO Box 50, York. (0904 29241)

Royal Association for Disability and Rehabilitation, 25 Mortimer Street, London W1. (01-637 5400)

Scottish Information Service for the Disabled, 18-19 Claremont Street, Edinburgh. (031 556 3892)

Society of Compassionate Friends, 10 Woodways, Watford, Hertfordshire. (92 24279)

SPOD, Committee on Sexual and Personal Relationships of the Disabled, Brook House, 2-16 Torrington Place, London WC1E 7HN.

Rudolf Steiner Special Schools and Homes Information Centre, Claverley Cottage, Lubbock Road, Chislehurst, Kent BR7 5LA.

Toy Libraries Association, Seabrook House, Wyllyots Manor, Darkes Lane, Potters Bar, Hertfordshire EN6 5HC. (0707 44571)

Voluntary Council for Handicapped Children, 8 Wakley Street, London EC1V 7QE. (01-278 9441)

3. Addresses in the United States of America

The following have been taken from the *Directory of National Information Sources on Handicapping Conditions and Related Services* published by the Department of Health, Education and Welfare, Washington, DC 20201.

Academy of Rehabilitative Audiology, Dept of Communication, 325 Derby Hall, Ohio State University, Columbus, OH 43210. (614-422-8207) Membership is open to qualified professionals but the inquiry service is open to all.

Adventures in Movement for the Handicapped, 945 Danbury Road, Dayton, OH 45420. (513-294-4611) The purpose is to provide movement education for children with handicaps, including the emotionally disturbed.

Aid to Adoption of Special Kids, 3530 Grand Avenue, Suite 202, Oakland, CA 94610. (415-451-1748)

Alexander Graham Bell Association for the Deaf, 3417 Volta Place, Washington, DC 20007. (202-337-5220)

Allergy Foundation of America, 801 Second Avenue, New York, NY 10017. (212-684-7875) All allergic diseases are served, including asthma.

American Academy for Cerebral Palsy, 1255 New Hampshire Avenue NW. Washington, DC 20036. (202-659-8251)

American Academy on Mental Retardation, 916 64th Avenue East, Tacoma, WA 98424. (206-922-5859) An organization composed of professionals engaged in research, with an inquiry service open to all.

American Alliance for Health, Physical Education and Recreation Information and Research Utilization Center, 1201 16th Street NW, Washington, DC 20036. (202-833-5547) For the collection and dissemination of activities and research connected with various handicapping conditions.

American Association for the Education of the Severely/Profoundly Handicapped, 1600 W. Armory Way, Seattle, WA 98119. (206-283-5055)

American Association on Mental Deficiency, 5101 Wisconsin Avenue NW, Washington, DC 20016. (202-686-5400)

American Association of Psychiatric Services for Children, 1701 18th Street NW, Washington, DC 20009. (202-332-7071) A membership association with an inquiry service open to all.

American Association of Workers for the Blind, 1511 K Street, Washington, DC 20005. (202-347-1559)

American Camping Association, Bradford Woods, Martinsville, IN 46151. (317-342-8456) Provides information about camps for handicapped individuals.

American Cancer Society, 777 Third Avenue, New York, NY 10017. (212-371-2900)

American Cleft Palate Association, 331 Salt Hall, University of Pittsburgh, Pittsburgh, PA 15261. (412-681-9620)

American Council of the Blind, 1211 Connecticut Avenue NW, Suite 506, Washington, DC 20036. (202-833-1251)

American Diabetes Association, 600 Fifth Avenue, New York, NY 10020. (212-541-4310)

American Foundation for the Blind, Inc., 15 W. 16th Street, New York, NY 10011. (212-924-0420)

American Heart Association, 7320 Greenville Avenue, Dallas, TX 75231. (214-750-5414)

American Lung Association, 1740 Broadway, New York, NY 10019. (212-245-8000)

American Printing House for the Blind, 1839 Frankfort Avenue, Louisville, KY 40206. (502-895-2405)

American Speech and Hearing Association, 10801 Rockville Pike, Rockville, MD 20852. (301-897-5700)

Amputee Shoe and Glove Exchange, 1115 Langford, College Station, TX 77840. (713-845-4016)

Association for Education of the Visually Handicapped, 919 Walnut Street, 4th Floor, Philadelphia, PA 19107. (215-923-7555)

Better Hearing Institute, 1430 K Street NW, Suite 800, Washington, DC 20005. (202-638-7577)

Center for Innovation in Teaching the Handicapped, University of Indiana, 2805 E. Tenth Street, Bloomington, IN 47401. (812-337-5847)

Centre for Sickle Cell Disease, 2121 Georgia Avenue NW, Washington, DC 20059. (202-636-7930)

Closer Look Information Center, 1201 16th Street NW, Washington, DC 20036. (202-833-4163) An information center on educational and other matters.

Communications Foundation, 600 New Hampshire Avenue NW, Washington, DC 20037. (202-333-0800) Dedicated to the application of modern technology to handicaps in human communication.

Cooley's Anemia Blood and Research Foundation for Children, Inc., 647 Franklin Avenue, Garden City, NY 11530. (516-747-2155)

Council for Exceptional Children Information Services, 1920 Association Drive, Reston, VA 22091. (703-620-3660)

Cystic Fibrosis Foundation, 3379 Peachtree Road NE, Atlanta, GA 30326. (404-262-1100)

Deafness Research Foundation, 366 Madison Avenue, New York, NY 10017. (212-682-3737)

Down's Syndrome Congress, 118 Paloma Drive, San Antonio, TX 78212.

Epilepsy Foundation of America, 1828 L Street NW, Washington, DC 20036. (202-293-2930)

Gessell Institute of Child Development, 310 Prospect Street, New Haven, CT 06511. (203-777-3481) Serving children with sensory impairments and learning disabilities.

Human Growth Foundation, Maryland Academy of Science Building, 601 Light Street, Baltimore, MD 21230. (612-831-2780)

International Association of Parents of the Deaf, 814 Thayer Avenue, Silver Spring, MD 20910. (310-585-5400)

John Tracy Clinic, 806 W. Adams Blvd, Los Angeles, CA 90007. (213-748-5481) An educational center for deaf children and their parents.

Joseph P. Kennedy Jr Foundation, 1701 K Street NW, Washington, DC 20006. (202-331-1731) For the study of mental retardation and its treatment.

Juvenile Diabetes Foundation, 23 E. 26th Street, New York, NY 10010. (212-689-7868)

Leukemia Society of America, 211 E. 43rd Street, New York, NY 10017. (212-573-8484)

Linguistics Research Laboratory, Gallaudet College, Florida Avenue and Seventh Street NE, Washington, DC 20002. (202-447-0707) Concerned with the language of deaf persons.

Lions International, York and Cermak Roads, Oak Brook, IL 60521. (312-986-1700)

Little People of America, PO Box 126, Owatonna, MN 55060. (507-451-1320) A voluntary organization of dwarfs.

Mental Disability Legal Resource Center, 1800 M Street NW, Washington DC, 20036. (202-331-2240)

Mental Health Law Project, 1220 19th Street NW, Suite 300, Washington, DC 20036. (202-467-5730)

Muscular Dystrophy Association Inc., 810 Seventh Avenue, New York, NY 10019. (212-586-0808)

National Association of the Deaf, 814 Thayer Avenue, Silver Spring, MD 20910. (301-587-1788)

National Association for Hearing and Speech Action, 814 Thayer Avenue, Silver Spring, MD 20910. (301-588-5242)

National Association for Mental Health Inc., 1800 N. Kent Street, Arlington, VA 22209. (703-528-6405)

National Association for Visually Handicapped, 305 E. 24th Street, 17-C, New York, NY 10010. (212-889-3141)

National Center for a Barrier Free Environment, 8401 Connecticut Avenue, Washington, DC 20015. (703-620-2731)

National Center for Law and the Deaf, Gallaudet College, Florida Avenue and Seventh Street NE, Washington, DC 20002. (202-447-0445)

National Center for Law and the Handicapped, 1235 N. Eddy Street, South Bend, IN 46617. (219-288-4751)

National Easter Seal Society for Crippled Children and Adults, 2023 W. Ogden Avenue, Chicago, IL 60612. (312-243-8400)

National Epilepsy League, 6 N. Michigan Avenue, Chicago, IL 60602. (312-332-6888)

National Foundation of Dentistry for the Handicapped, 1211 Broadway, Suite 5, Boulder, CO 80302. (303-443-7920)

National Genetics Foundation, 9 West 57th Street, New York, NY 10019. (212-759-4432)

National Hemophilia Foundation, 25 W. 39th Street, New York, NY 10018. (212-869-9740)

National Kidney Foundation, 116 E. 27th Street, New York, NY 10016. (212-889-2210)

National Paraplegia Foundation, 333 N. Michigan Avenue, Chicago, IL 60601. (312-346-4779)

National Society for Autistic Children, 306 31st Street, Huntingdon, WV 25702. (304-697-2638)

National Tay-Sachs and Allied Diseases Association, 122 E. 42nd Street, New York, NY 10017. (212-661-2780)

National Tuberous Sclerosis Association, PO Box 159, Laguna Beach, CA 92652. (714-494-8900)

North American Riding for the Handicapped Association Inc., PO Box 100, Ashburn, VA 22011. (703-777-3540)

Rubella Project, Roosevelt Hospital, 428 W. 59th Street, New York, NY 10019. (212-554-6565)

Sertoma Foundation, Sertoma Centers for Communicative Disorders, 750 Montclair Road, Birmingham, AL 35213. (205-591-6047)

Sex Information and Education Council of the U.S., 137-155 N. Franklin Street, Hempstead, NY 11550. (516-483-3033)

Society for the Rehabilitation of the Facially Disfigured, 550 First Avenue, New York, NY 10016. (212-679-1534)

Spina Bifida Association of America, 209 Shiloh Drive, Madison, WI 53705. (608-836-8969)

Trace Research and Development Center for the Severely Communicatively Handicapped, 1500 Highland Avenue, Room 314, Madison, WI 53706. (608-262-6966)

United Cerebral Palsy Associations Inc., 66 E. 34th Street, New York, NY 10016. (212-481-6300)

Name index

Vernon, D.T.A., 5, 33, 38
Vernon, P.E., 63
Vinstainer, M.A., 36

Ward, Timothy, 191
Willis, Thomas, 98
Wills, Doris, 139

Wing, Lorna, 78, 81
Wolfer, J.A., 36
Wonnacott, Linda, 6
Woodward, J., 40
World Health Organization, 123

Yudkin, Simon, 150, 157

Subject index